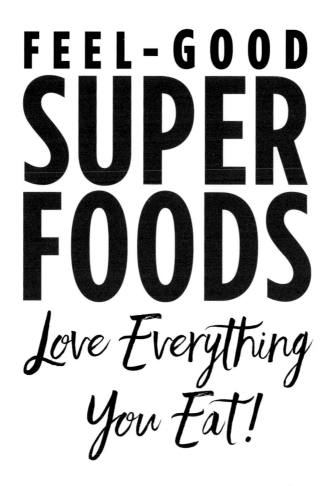

FEEL-GOOD
SUPER
FOODS

Love Everything You Eat!

TABITHA GRACE ALTERMAN

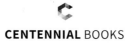

CENTENNIAL BOOKS

CENTENNIAL BOOKS

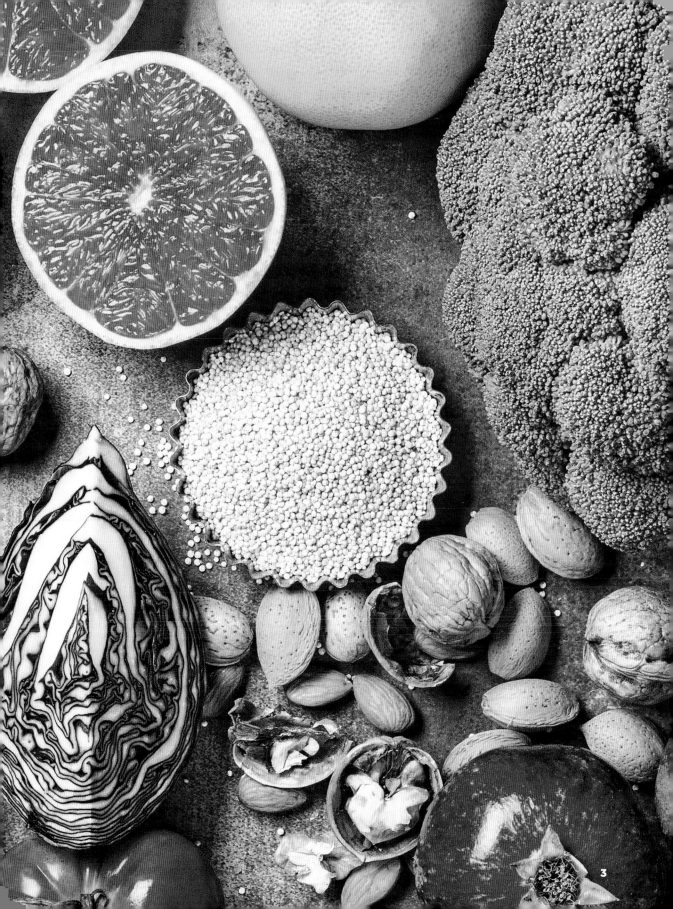

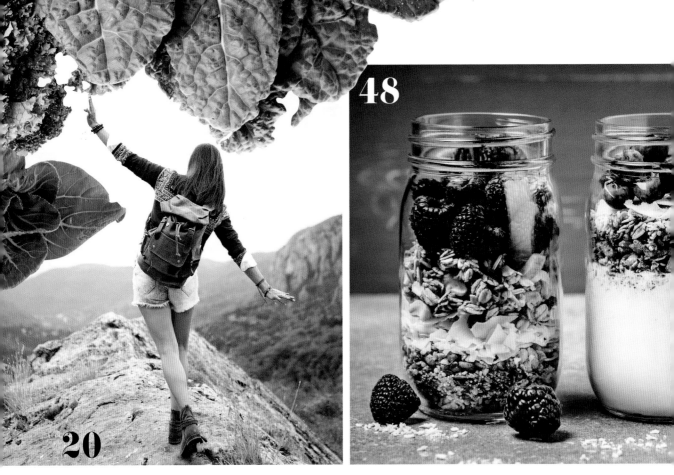

48

20

Contents

PART 1
**The Basics
of Healthy Eating**

08 Why Superfoods?
Delicious ingredients to
elevate your health.

14 What to Eat Every Day
Follow this dietary blueprint
for better health.

**20 8 Ways Healthy Foods
Can Change Your Life**
Why your diet makes a big
difference.

24 Deficient Nutrition
Get crucial missing nutrients
back into your food.

**28 How Superfoods
Changed My Life**
Secrets from a leading
cookbook author.

30 Eat Well for Life
Simple ideas to improve your
diet one step at a time.

**36 Shopping Tips for
Affordable Goodness**
How to eat well without
busting your budget.

40 Smart Swaps
Clean up your grocery list
with healthier substitutes.

44 Sneaky Nutrient Boosts
Clever ideas to get the best
ingredients into every meal.

48 Nutrition Myths—Busted!
Separate fact from fiction to
get to a healthier you.

**54 "Health Foods" That
Aren't So Healthy**
Watch out for these sneaky
dietary imposters.

58 Foods That Help You Heal
Reduce illness and feel
better with these options.

62 Superfoods, Super Mood
Improve energy, focus,
mood, sleep and more.

**64 Fun Facts About
Healthy Foods**
Surprising tidbits about
what's in your diet.

PART 2
A—Z Superfoods Guide

70 Açai Berry
72 Artichoke
74 Avocado
76 Barley
78 Black Bean
**80 Blueberry and
More Berries**

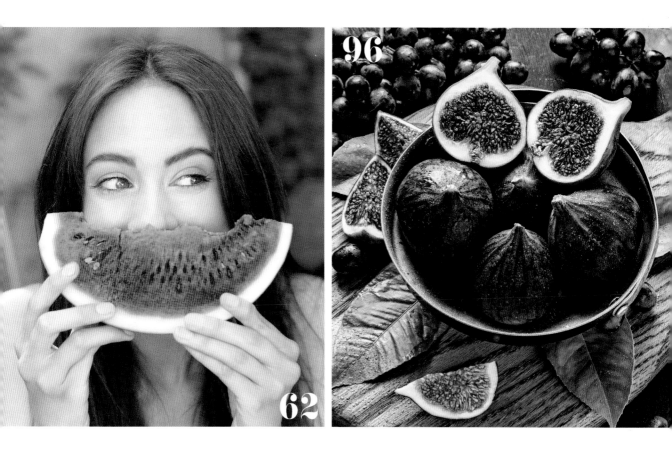

84	**Coconut**	106	**Hemp Seed and Flaxseed**	156	**Rosemary**
86	**Coffee**	108	**Horseradish**	158	**Sardine**
88	**Cheese**	110	**In-Season Veggies**	160	**Sauerkraut and Kimchi**
90	**Dark Chocolate**	112	**Jalapeño and Spicy Peppers**	162	**Tea**
92	**Date**	116	**Kale**	164	**Tomato**
94	**Eggplant**	118	**Lemon**	166	**Turmeric**
96	**Fig**	120	**Lentil**	168	**Undersea Superfood**
98	**Garbanzo Bean**	122	**Macadamia Nut**	170	**Vinegar**
100	**Garlic**	124	**Mushroom**	172	**Walnut and Other Nuts**
102	**Grass-Fed Meat**	128	**Mussel**	176	**Wild Rice**
104	**Greens**	130	**Nettle**	178	**Wild Salmon**
		132	**Olive Oil and More Oils**	180	**Xtra Superfoods**
		136	**Onion**	182	**Yogurt**
		138	**Organic Egg**	184	**Zucchini**
		140	**Plum**	186	**Index**
		142	**Potato, Roots and Tubers**		
		146	**Pumpkin Seed**		
		148	**Quality Dairy**		
		150	**Quinoa and Ancient Grains**		
		154	**Raspberry**		

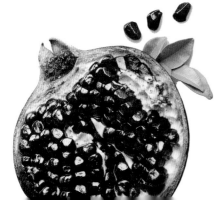

PART 1

The Basics of Healthy Eating

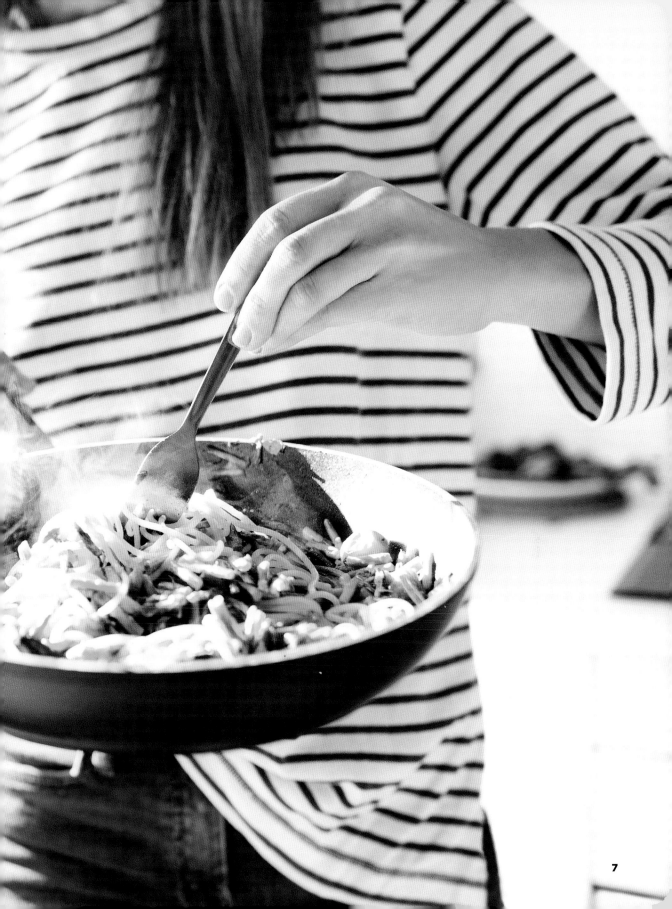

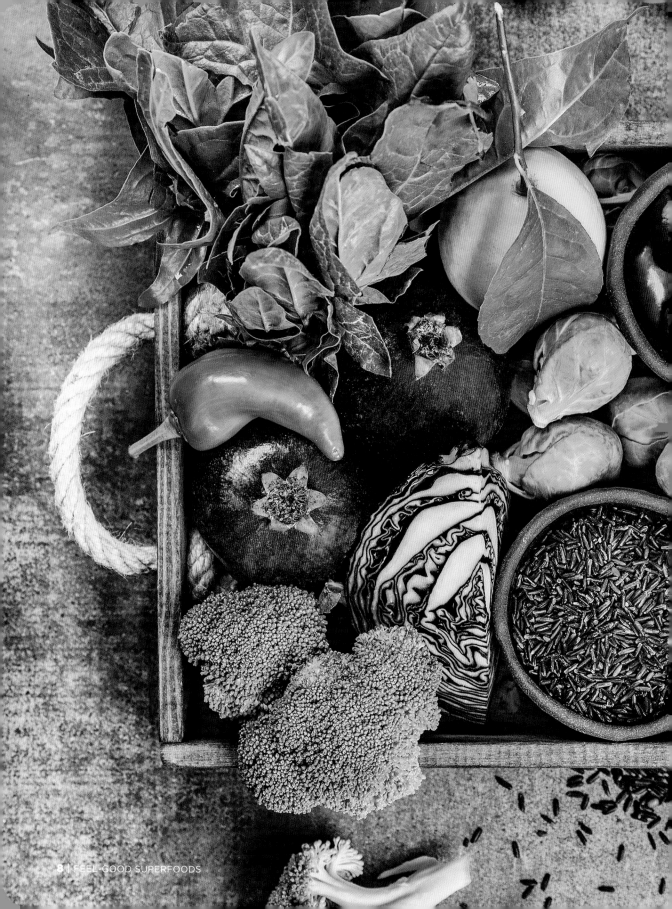

Why Superfoods?

These delicious and potent ingredients elevate health, happiness, mood and energy.

At its simplest, the concept of superfoods encompasses the whole range of fresh produce available everywhere. That means fruits and vegetables, of course, but there's so much more. Superfoods also include tons of culinary herbs, spices, mushrooms and other wild edibles likely to be available near you. If we all started cooking and eating more of these fruits and veggies, herbs and spices, we'd be well on our way to wellness. Go a step further and be sure to consume the widest possible *variety* of these foods, and we're even closer to optimum health.

Besides these commonplace foods, we now have access to super-nutritious edibles coming from all over the planet, including coffee, tea, wine and fermented beverages; wild-caught seafood; grass-fed meat; butter, milk and cheese; and a number of exotic-sounding roots and powders. In a varied diet composed largely of whole foods, we don't need to be overly concerned about the intake of specific nutrients (or calories). But if we sprinkle in some of the most potent medicines from nature—superfoods—we maximize the potential food has to enhance our lives. Why wouldn't we manage whatever we can when it comes to living our best lives? Read on for more reasons to think super.

1
Nutrient Density

Superfoods are super, either because they contain unique compounds with specific, well-researched and documented health benefits (such as the ability to slow tumor growth, assist with weight loss, or improve cholesterol levels), or because they're especially nutrient-dense per calorie. Some people have a narrow definition of superfoods that doesn't include foods rich in fat, protein and carbohydrates. However, there are super versions of these foods too. I have included both *nutrient-dense* foods and particularly healthy, *energy-dense* foods in this guide. I've focused mainly on widely available, everyday foods with super properties, but hopefully you'll also encounter some new items to love. All these foods have the potential to dramatically upgrade overall health, vitality, mood and energy levels.

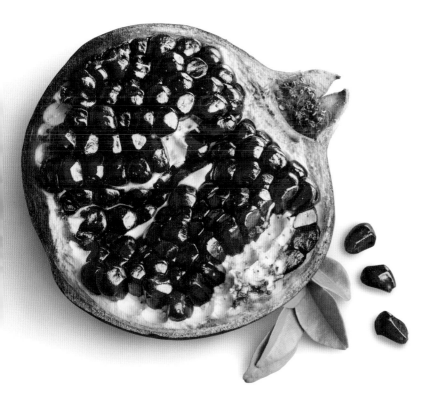

2
Food as Medicine

Superfoods have high concentrations of vitamins and minerals, all in an enticing array of colors and flavors. (In fact, rich colors often are an indicator of nutrient content and deep flavor.) Superfoods deliver extra-healthy versions of the energy molecules our bodies use as fuel. They also boast high levels of powerful phytonutrients (plant nutrients) that prevent all kinds of disease. The majority of medicines were discovered in plants, after all.

These critical nutrients—many of which are deficient in today's diet (more about that on the next page)—can help lower blood pressure and cholesterol; improve blood sugar, mood, memory, concentration, sleep and critical thinking; reduce stress, anxiety and depression; and help you lose weight and feel satisfied and energized all day long!

Open your mind and pantry to superfoods, and you'll be feeling and looking great in short order. You'll probably also get a kick out of having something different to try when it comes to the day-in, day-out task of feeding yourself and your family. Best of all, you'll find some new foods to love—reason enough to give them a try.

3 Superfoods Can Be Simple

Besides being powerhouse disease fighters and energy boosters, superfood ingredients are also temptingly delicious and often quite easy to use. Many of the superfoods included here, such as beans, greens, eggs and mushrooms, are commonplace and relatively inexpensive.

Incorporating superfoods into your diet does not need to be complicated. Sometimes it's just a matter of sprinkling a new ingredient onto one of your favorite dishes (think berries in your cereal and oatmeal; hemp seeds or seaweed on a salad); or swapping out one of the less-healthy ingredients in your pantry (milk chocolate) for its higher-caliber version (dark chocolate).

Fresh, in-season, nutrient-supercharged tomatoes and asparagus are wonderful with just a sprinkle of salt. Cancer-cell-killing broccoli and Brussels sprouts need only a quick brushing with olive oil and a little time in a hot oven to reach their peak flavor potential. Even cooking fish like salmon, sardines and mussels is far easier than you probably think. Many of the superfoods in this guide can simply be enjoyed fresh and raw, or blended with other superfoods into a nutritious and filling smoothie.

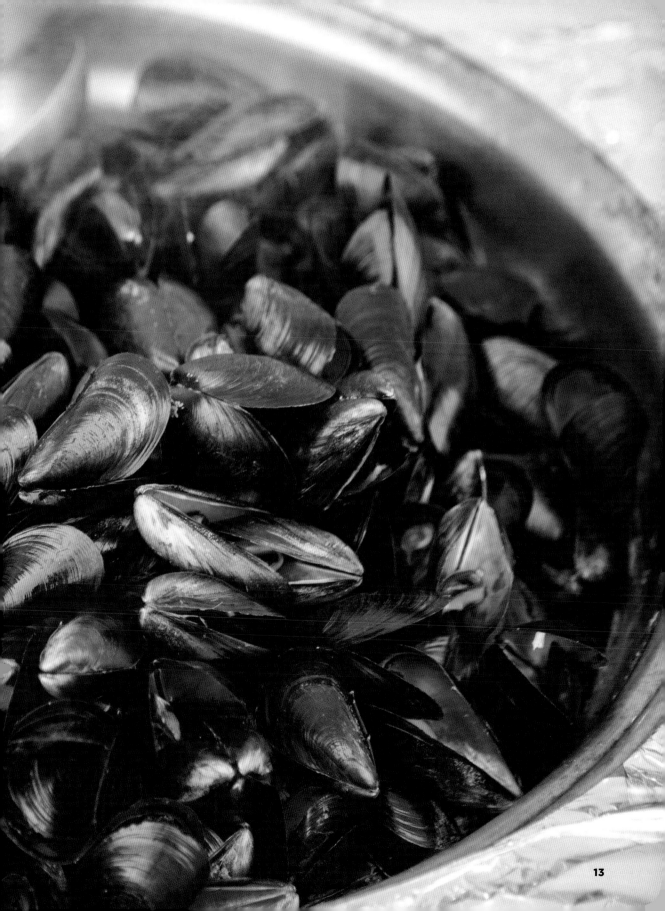

What to Eat Every Day

To take control of your health—and enjoy a fuller, more pleasurable life—it's essential to follow a plan. Here's a daily blueprint that guarantees success.

Fruits, veggies and whole grains contain phytochemicals that give them color (and help fight disease!).

That co-worker who eats the exact same lunch (spinach, salmon, vinaigrette) every day, or that friend who always orders a kale salad? Believe it or not, their diets may not be as healthy as they think. While leafy greens definitely deserve their glowing-health halo, it's just as important to eat a variety of foods as any single thing, no matter how nutritious it may be.

"You can eat a lot of kale, but then you're missing out on other micronutrients," says Joel Fuhrman, MD, whose most recent book is *Fast Food Genocide*. Instead, he recommends branching out into an array of whole, natural foods that work together for optimal energy and well-being. "This will ensure you're getting the vitamins, minerals, antioxidants, phytochemicals and other micronutrients that protect against disease—especially cancer, heart disease and dementia," he says.

The USDA recommends eating five to nine servings of fruits and vegetables per day.

Follow the Rainbow

An easy way to make sure you're eating a diverse diet is to consume a literal "rainbow" of plant foods, from deep purple and blue (red cabbage, blueberries) to white (onions, navy beans, cauliflower). This kaleidoscope provides the nutrients that "allow us to enjoy life into our later years and not age like everyone else," says Fuhrman, who has launched an Eat to Live Retreat in San Juan Capistrano, California, to help people reverse disease and lose weight on his Nutritarian Diet. "In all the Blue Zones, which are these long-living societies where you see the most centenarians, 90 percent of their diet is unrefined plants," Fuhrman says—an amount he recommends to his patients.

Where's the Beef?

But 90 percent plants? Many Americans wonder how they'd ever get enough protein eating a diet that's almost entirely fruits and vegetables. The truth is, you don't need a whole porterhouse steak or half a chicken to get an adequate amount of protein. In fact, "the maximum amount of animal products you include in your diet should be less than 5 percent, which is under 20 ounces a week," Fuhrman insists. Instead, you can get all the protein you need from plant foods—some of which are even higher in protein per calorie than meat, he says. "We know that eating high-protein animal products causes more deaths from cancer, while high-protein plant foods reduce the risk."

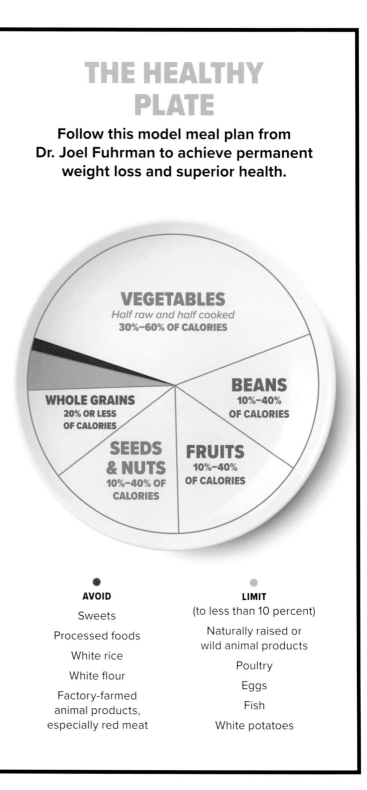

THE HEALTHY PLATE

Follow this model meal plan from Dr. Joel Fuhrman to achieve permanent weight loss and superior health.

VEGETABLES
Half raw and half cooked
30%–60% OF CALORIES

BEANS
10%–40% OF CALORIES

WHOLE GRAINS
20% OR LESS OF CALORIES

SEEDS & NUTS
10%–40% OF CALORIES

FRUITS
10%–40% OF CALORIES

● **AVOID**

Sweets

Processed foods

White rice

White flour

Factory-farmed animal products, especially red meat

○ **LIMIT**
(to less than 10 percent)

Naturally raised or wild animal products

Poultry

Eggs

Fish

White potatoes

SEND IN THE G-BOMBS

To remind us to eat the variety of superfoods our bodies need on a regular basis, Fuhrman came up with an acronym: G-BOMBS, which stands for greens, beans, onions, mushrooms, berries and seeds. Here's why they're so important.

GREENS

Because they contain only 100 calories per pound, they fill you up with minimal calories. Eat a large salad with some cruciferous veggies every day.

17

BERRIES

Whether your favorite color is blue, black or strawberry red, berries are linked to a reduced risk of diabetes, cancer and dementia. Eat three fresh fruits a day, including a cup of berries.

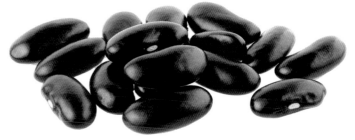

MUSHROOMS

Consuming just 10 grams—the size of your thumb—of cooked mushrooms every day can lower your breast cancer risk by 64 percent, according to a study of Asian women.

BEANS

Eat a half cup of beans every day. "In the Nurses' Health Study, women who ate beans three times a week had a 26 percent lower rate of breast cancer," Fuhrman notes.

SEEDS

This category includes flax, hemp, chia and sunflower seeds as well as nuts. Both supply unique micronutrients, including plant sterols that reduce cholesterol levels and fight heart disease. Eat an ounce a day of nuts or seeds.

ONIONS

"Eat a little raw onion or some scallions every day," Fuhrman advises. They contain valuable organosulfate compounds, which target cancer cells.

8 Ways Healthy Foods Can Change Your Life

Whatever your wellness goals—from glowing skin to a sharper mind to the stamina of the Energizer Bunny— what you eat holds the key.

1

PROVIDE NOURISHMENT

Healthy foods boost energy, build strength and may even create a happier life for you and your family. A study conducted at the University of Pennsylvania linked good nutrition with positive social development in children.

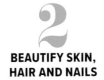

2

BEAUTIFY SKIN, HAIR AND NAILS

Radiant skin, shiny hair and strong, shapely nails show your inner health to the world. Foods high in beta-carotene—papaya, sweet potatoes, carrots—get skin glowing, while those with biotin, a vitamin found in eggs, milk and bananas, can help stop hair loss and strengthen brittle nails.

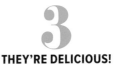

3

THEY'RE DELICIOUS!

In case you need another reason to eat a healthy diet: It tastes amazing! Once you start eating nutritious whole foods, processed and fast foods will taste overly salty, greasy and thoroughly unappetizing.

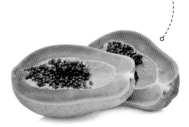

You probably know that eating more vegetables, whole fruits and lean protein can help you lose weight. But a diet rich in superfoods can also have a positive effect on so many other things in your life: It can protect you from getting colds and the flu this winter—and from getting dementia decades from now. It can improve digestion, prevent cardiovascular disease and diabetes. And last but not least, it can give you beautiful skin, hair and nails. And you don't have to make drastic changes! Even little tweaks, like swapping one serving of meat for beans, or eating an additional piece of fruit a day, can make a difference. More good news? It's never too late to take that first step.

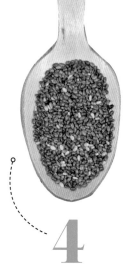

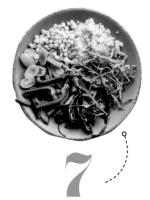

4
AID DIGESTION

If gas, bloating, heartburn, nausea, constipation or diarrhea are part of your everyday life, you can rehab your GI tract with better eating habits. A diet that's high in fiber and rich in whole grains, vegetables, legumes and fruits has been shown to keep food moving through your digestive tract, helping to prevent or treat digestive conditions and irritable bowel syndrome.

5
BOOST IMMUNITY

A recent German study found that the immune system reacts to a high-fat and high-calorie diet the same way it does to a bacterial infection, creating inflammation. On the other hand, antioxidant-rich foods can switch on genes that fight off bacteria—as well as cell damage, disease and the common cold.

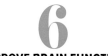

6
IMPROVE BRAIN FUNCTION

Food for thought isn't just an expression: Certain foods can actually sharpen your thinking and prevent cognitive decline. Research at the Center for Brain Plasticity at the University of Illinois at Urbana-Champaign has linked high blood levels of omega-3 fatty acids with improved cognitive function. Fatty fish like salmon, trout, sardines, mackerel, tuna and herring are loaded with omega-3s.

7
OFFER HEALING POWERS

Want to ditch the insulin and toss the statins? A plant-based diet that is low in calories is the most effective for reversing diabetes while simultaneously treating cardiovascular disease, according to a 2017 study in the *Journal of Geriatric Cardiology*.

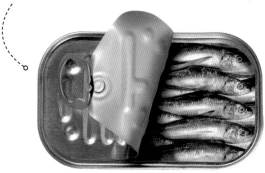

8
INCREASE LONGEVITY

Want to be around for your 80th, 85th, 90th—even your 100th—birthday? Healthy eating is your best bet. A 2017 study published in the *New England Journal of Medicine* found that people who added some wholesome foods over time—even if they didn't commit to a complete diet makeover—improved their chances of living longer.

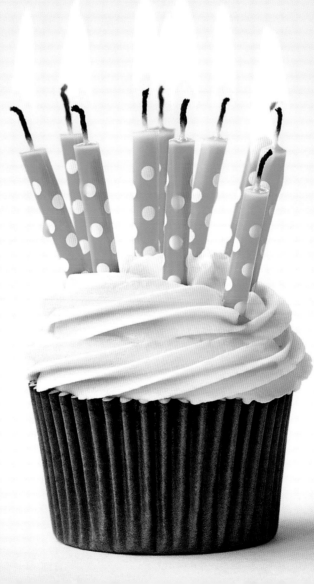

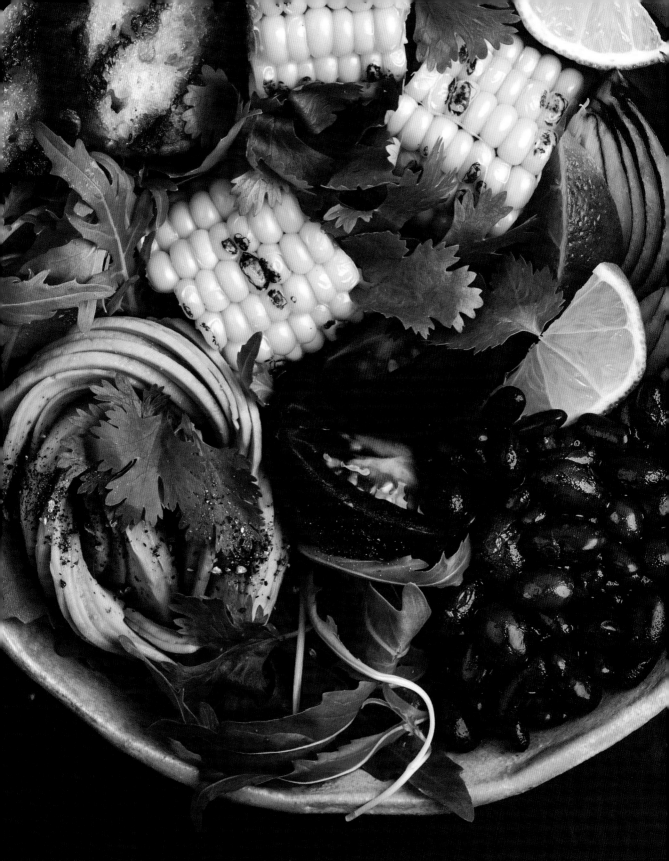

Deficient Nutrition

Most Americans are undernourished, no matter how much they eat. Learn how to get crucial missing nutrients back into your food.

Lack of variety in our diets is a significant problem for many Americans. According to Yale-trained physician Aviva Romm, at least 80 percent of us do not get the nutrients we need for basic health. The USDA examines nutrient deficiency every five years, and its most recent analysis revealed that Americans are deficient in 10 critical nutrients. Americans are so extraordinarily deficient in four of these—calcium, dietary fiber, potassium and vitamin D— that the USDA classifies this as

posing a substantial public health concern. In addition, females under age 50 aren't getting enough iron. Folate, magnesium and vitamins A, C and E are classified as "underconsumed nutrients"—we're getting some, but not enough.

To correct these dangerous trends, the USDA and nutrition experts encourage us to eat nutrient-dense foods. By doing so, we can prevent many kinds of chronic disease, improve physical fitness and overall wellness, and even increase our brain

capacity. In a 2015 study from the Australian National University, participants who ate the most nutrient-dense foods over four years developed millions more brain cells than those who didn't. We all need to eat a wider variety of vegetables, fruits, legumes, whole grains, nuts and seeds to help correct these deficiencies. Check out how these and other superfoods— the most nutrient-dense foods there are—can increase your intake of the specific nutrients you may be missing.

Superfood Sources

CALCIUM

Calcium is essential to bone health, memory and critical thinking, and low levels can cause anxiety, depression, irritability and weight gain. Dairy is an excellent source, but many greens also contain absorbable calcium. (We also need sufficient vitamin D, potassium and magnesium to process calcium.)

Best Sources

Dairy

Greens (especially kale, collards, turnip, mustard and bok choy)

Kelp

Cabbage

Sardines

Nuts

MAGNESIUM

Magnesium, which is increasingly deficient in our soils, plays critical roles in improving memory, blood sugar, brain and heart health. This calming mineral also relaxes the mind, muscles and nerves, improves sleep, reduces anxiety, and is used to treat clinical depression.

Best Sources

Beans

Greens

Nuts and seeds

Fatty fish

Papaya

Vegetables

Whole grains

Blackstrap molasses

FOLATE

Folate helps prevent birth defects, heart disease, dementia and cancer. It also improves memory, pleasure and clarity of thinking, and is critical for the production of DNA and many brain chemicals. Folate is light-sensitive, so using fresh ingredients is key. Also, naturally occurring folate (in food) is more effective than folic acid supplementation.

Best Sources

Greens (especially spinach and kale)

Legumes

Vegetables

Pastured eggs

Chicken liver

IRON

Iron is the nutrient that most people in the world lack. The brain needs iron for processing speed, memory, and the ability to feel pleasure. It's especially important for brains to get enough iron when they are developing. Iron is also a critical player in our bodies' natural detox systems. (Note that we absorb more iron from animal foods than from plants.)

Best Sources

Grass-fed meat

Shellfish

Pumpkin and sesame seeds

Greens

Dark chocolate

Dried fruit

FIBER

Dietary fiber is critical to keep your digestive system operating well, and it is the food source for the healthy microbes in our gut. High fiber improves cholesterol ratios, and helps maintain stable blood sugar levels and healthy weight. Fiber also reduces inflammation. Low fiber can slow brain growth and cause mood problems and depression.

Best Sources

Vegetables (especially broccoli, cauliflower and greens)

Fruit (especially raspberries)

Legumes

Tempeh

# of Missing Nutrients

POTASSIUM

Potassium helps prevent bone loss and kidney stones, and counteracts the negative effects of getting too much salt (which is easy to do if you eat processed foods). Potassium is also important to nerve and muscle health. To get more potassium, you'll have to eat more plant foods. Also note that caffeine can interfere with potassium absorption.

Best Sources

Beans

Coconut water

Fruits (especially bananas)

Vegetables (especially artichokes, avocados and squash)

Greens

Mushrooms

VITAMIN A

Vitamin A is vital for mood, memory and making new brain cells. It also promotes vision, healthy skin and immunity, and helps prevent dementia and cancer. Pigments called carotenoids in certain foods, such as carrots and peppers, can be converted into vitamin A in our bodies (especially from orange and yellow foods). The only source of readily usable vitamin A is animal fat.

Best Sources

Grass-fed meat (especially chicken liver), eggs and dairy

Shellfish

Orange and yellow plants

Greens (especially mustard)

VITAMIN C

Antioxidant vitamin C helps us grow and repair blood vessels, bones, teeth, skin and various tissues of the body. It also helps fight premature aging, cancer, heart disease and other illnesses. To get the most vitamin C, eat produce raw. Many studies have also shown that organic fruits and vegetables contain more vitamin C than conventional produce.

Best Sources

Fruit (especially berries, citrus and papaya)

Greens

Vegetables (especially broccoli, cauliflower, cabbage, peppers and tomatoes)

VITAMIN D

Vitamin D is important for bone health and immunity, and is critical for brain health. Low levels are linked with many mental disorders. We make vitamin D when our skin is exposed to the sun, so this may explain the prevalence of seasonal affective disorder. We need fat in our diet to be able to absorb vitamin D, and we need vitamin D in our bodies to be able to absorb calcium.

Best Sources

Grass-fed meat (especially pork ribs), eggs (especially the yolks) and dairy products

Mushrooms (if exposed to sun)

Wild-caught salmon, sardines and trout

VITAMIN E

There are eight different forms of vitamin E, which makes another good case for eating a variety of whole foods. Vitamin E protects brain cells and can decrease cognitive decline and slow the onset of Alzheimer's. It also helps prevent heart disease and cancer. Low vitamin E is correlated with clinical depression. Vitamin E also keeps your skin glowing. This nutrient is much more powerful in food than in supplements.

Best Sources

Avocado

Nuts and seeds

Pastured eggs

Greens (especially spinach)

Olives and extra-virgin olive oil

27

How Superfoods Changed My Life

Julie Morris, author of five superfoods cookbooks, has energy all day long—thanks to nature's most amazing foods.

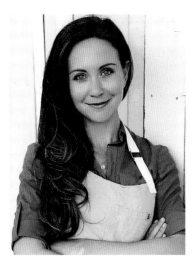

What are superfoods?

The most nutrient-dense, benefit-rich foods in nature. The key is the ratio of micronutrients per calorie. These are the vitamins, minerals, antioxidants and phytochemicals we need in small quantities, yet are essential. They're also the components most lacking in our diet. Looking at food this way, it's clear which foods rise to the top. It's not that other foods don't offer benefits. It's just that superfoods, such as leafy greens, berries, super seeds like chia and hemp, and medicinal mushrooms like shiitake, offer so much *more*.

How did you come to start enjoying superfoods?

At 20, I was suffering from allergies, inability to feel rested after sleep, low energy in the afternoon, slow recovery after exercise, and more. I felt awful, day after day. Not having luck at the doctor, I took matters into my own hands and began researching energy foods. I read about healing foods revered in their native cultures and decided to try a couple—maca root and goji berries. I gave myself a month to be a guinea pig. The experience was life-changing. In addition to feeling a *huge* shift in energy, it was the first time I became aware of how good I could feel after eating. (Normally I experienced the opposite!) I've been hooked since.

How super are superfoods, really? Is there any proof?

Using nutrient density as a baseline to make better food choices, there's all the proof in the world. Take chia seeds. They contain five times more calcium than milk, three times more iron than spinach, eight times more omega-3s than salmon, and numerous other nutrients. That's incredibly effective, "super" healthy eating. Superfoods are increasingly being studied in scientific circles, validating long-known health claims.

What has been your most significant dietary change?

I decided to try vegetarianism at 14 (I later became a vegan and still am). This was big for me, as my family was heavily reliant on animal products. Then, around the time I started eating superfoods, I became more conscious about eating clean. I ate so many processed foods I assumed were healthy because they were vegetarian—untrue. I refocused on whole, plant-based foods and ingredients, and made sure the few packaged foods I consumed included only ingredients I might also have in my own kitchen, which works as an effective grocery shopping credo.

And the most significant result of eating superfoods?

Energy. Not the crazed, four-cups-of-coffee kind, but the sustainable, I-can-do-more-with-my-day kind.

I'd love to hear about someone you've influenced.

One reader was passionate about staying active. She also used to skip breakfast, got frequent headaches and experienced mental fog. Her tipping point was contracting viral meningitis, which left her feeling too sick to do her favorite things. After reading *Superfood Smoothies*, she made one recipe each morning, slowly incorporated the ingredients into her cooking, and eliminated other foods after becoming aware of the way they made her feel. After two months, her health had transformed. In her words, "I can honestly say I have never felt so good! I can take on my day, feeling strong, having more focus and clarity, just feeling great!"

If you could only get a few exotic superfoods into your life, which would they be?

Spirulina, goji berries and any kind of medicinal mushroom. The longevity potential of these three is astounding.

Eat Well for Life

Try these simple ideas for improving your diet one step at a time.

Ideally, we would all eat whenever we are truly hungry, and enjoy the foods most likely to make us feel energized, happy and satiated. Establishing a healthy eating pattern can be difficult, however, if nutrition concepts are new to you and especially if you don't like to cook. But eating healthfully doesn't have to be about unusual ingredients or complicated cooking techniques. Nutrient-dense superfoods taste great, even when prepared simply. And there's no need for dieting when your diet is generally nutritious. If you have a solid baseline to return to, you can also occasionally splurge without much worry.

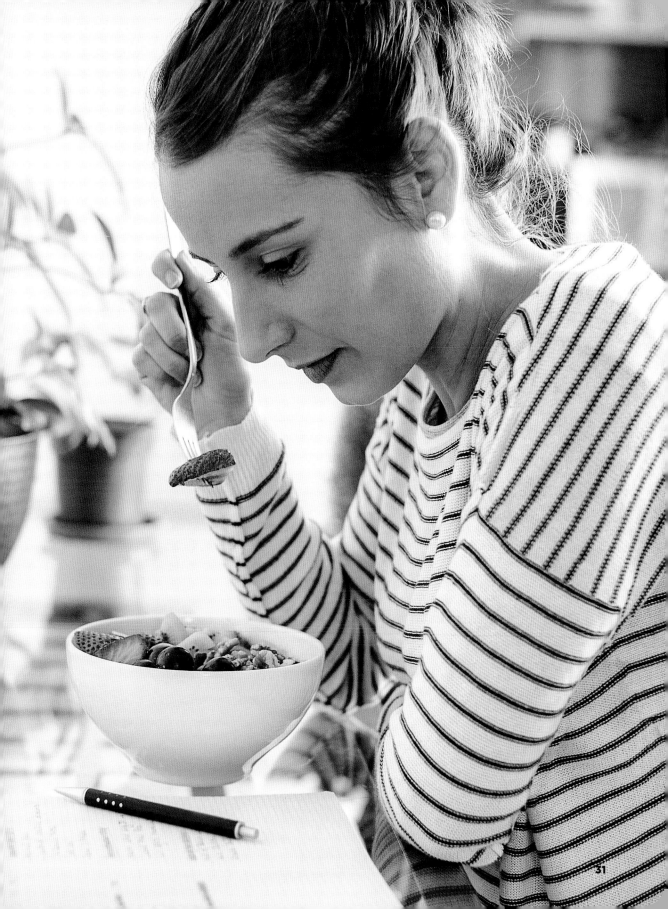

To Eat Well, Pay Attention

If you're trying to get into a new rhythm with food, it's important to pay close attention to how you feel—physically, emotionally and mentally—whenever you are craving specific foods and after you have eaten them. You can also notice what time of day it is, who you're with, where you are, how much sleep you've had, whether you feel stressed, and other factors you might not realize are affecting your diet. Your healthy and unhealthy eating patterns may become clearer than you'd guess when reflected upon this way.

The best way to pay attention is not to count calories, but instead to keep a food journal. Many studies show that this practice can help you lose excess weight and keep it off successfully. You don't need to get overly detailed. Just jot down what you notice before and after eating (up to a couple of hours afterward). Once you identify troublesome foods or patterns, make a plan to change

things one step at a time. Keep in mind that you may be used to (or addicted to) sugary, salty, starchy, fried or unnaturally flavored foods. Taste buds can change, but it usually takes at least a week. Be patient with yourself, and try plenty of new flavors in the meantime. Use this guide to find new tastes to try!

While you are attempting to notice and change patterns, it's helpful to avoid restaurants. Studies correlate restaurant eating with weight gain and an unhealthy cholesterol ratio. When we tune in to our bodies, we know what to eat, when and how much. And then we can simply enjoy eating.

Know What to Eat

You probably know that fruits and vegetables are good for you. Beyond that, it can be hard to know which foods to eat. You might have cravings for foods you know will not make you feel good. Or you might have health problems and wonder if food is a cause. Often, we end

up eating foods that are not nourishing because we need their quick energy.

Food journaling can help you figure all this out, but here is the basic idea of good nutrition: Eat a balanced diet composed of a variety—emphasis on variety—of whole, unprocessed foods. Focus on eating lots of plants (leaves, roots, fruits, nuts, seeds, legumes and whole grains). Choose high-quality proteins. Be sure to include satiating, healthy fats. For help determining how much of these foods to eat, keep reading!

Know When to Eat

We should eat whenever we're hungry, right? Sounds simple. But hunger is complex, and we're not all experts at deciphering hunger cues. Are we hungry because we're bored, or because it's 6 p.m., or because we're at a family gathering and food is just… there? When we have cravings for specific foods, are we hungry enough to eat vegetables or fruit? If not, it's a good clue that we may be craving that food for emotional reasons.

For some people, a big breakfast followed by two lighter meals is enough. Other people need healthy snacks between meals to keep their blood sugar in balance, or may operate best on several small meals a day. Try a few different approaches, and use your food journal to determine the eating schedule that gives you enough energy throughout the day, makes your body feel good, keeps you in a good mood, and sets you up for a great night of sleep. The following approach works well for

Don't Sabotage Yourself!

If you want to eat healthy, you need to get ready. If there's no healthy food in your house, you won't be able to eat it. If there's junk food around (processed and sugary foods, refined flour products), you'll grab it when your best intentions have vanished. Plan for quick, simple meals on busy nights. Use our A to Z Guide (starting on page 68) to help you shop for superfoods—start with whatever looks appealing, and don't get too fancy if you know you'll be short on time. Also think about times you'll need to have healthy options with you outside the home, such as at work. Avoid eating in the car or on the couch.

many people—it's a good place to start:

- As soon as you wake up, have a full glass of warm water with a squirt of lemon juice to promote hydration and healthy bowel movements.
- Make a breakfast composed mainly of protein, vegetables and a healthy fat. Include a small portion of whole grains if you tolerate them well. Try to incorporate a little of something fermented, such as yogurt or kimchi.
- Be sure you're hungry when you eat again. Waiting three hours is a good starting point. If you find yourself getting shaky, exhausted or irritable between meals, this may mean your blood sugar has dropped and small snacks are important for you.
- For lunch, eat plenty of greens, plus more colorful vegetables, quality protein and, again, some of that healthy fat. Also include a serving of starchy food (learn the differences between carb types on page 52).
- At dinner, go for some greens again, more veggies (remember you're trying to get around eight servings a day), more protein and fat, and another serving or two of slow carbs. Aim to finish eating a few hours before sleep.

Knowing when *not* to eat can be helpful, too. Recent studies have shown that fasting boosts metabolism, increases energy, and reduces the inflammation that leads to numerous diseases. For people with blood sugar issues, intense fasting will never work. One way to get some of the benefits of fasting is to simply make sure there are about 12 hours between your dinner (maybe 7 p.m.) and your breakfast (7 a.m.).

Know How Much to Eat

Many people don't know what appropriate portion sizes are, because restaurants have confused us. Often, we eat everything on the plate, beyond being satiated. Here are a few ways to manage portions: Eat slowly; try to clue in to feelings of fullness; use small plates and bowls; serve food and then put extras away before you sit down to eat; and begin meals by eating your most nutrient-dense foods first. Below you'll find portion recommendations for specific food groups.

Dairy If you tolerate dairy well, you can enjoy a serving at each meal. Consider a serving to be one cup of liquid dairy (yogurt, kefir) or an ounce or two of cheese. Always choose whole-fat dairy products. Full-fat dairy is correlated with a lower risk of gaining weight, and current nutrition science does not support recommendations to choose low-fat dairy products.

Fats Enjoy one or two tablespoons of high-quality fats in every meal, such as oils from avocado, coconut, olive, sesame, sunflower and walnut; butter and ghee from grass-fed animals; and lard and other animal fats from pastured livestock. If you feel the need for a snack between meals, be sure to make it one containing healthy fat.

Fermented Foods To build up your healthy gut flora to bolster your immune system, mood and more, use fermented seasonings such as soy sauce and vinegar. Try to include other fermented foods in each meal, too, such as sauerkraut, yogurt, sourdough bread, or brined olives and pickles.

Fruit A serving of small fruits, such as berries, is approximately half a cup. Apples, pears and other fruits eaten out of hand are considered to be a single serving. Enjoy a couple of servings of fruit per day, and skip the fruit juices.

Herbs and Spices Use fresh herbs and dried spices liberally. Add these nutrient powerhouses to all of your meals in abundance.

Legumes (beans, lentils and peas) Aim for half a cup at lunch and dinner. If your tummy tends to be sensitive to beans, see how you do with chickpeas and lentils, which most people can handle. Also eat plenty of fermented foods to improve digestion.

Meat, Seafood and Eggs
A couple of eggs or approximately four to six ounces of meat or fish will provide energy for a few hours, while keeping your blood sugar steady.

Mushrooms If you like earthy mushrooms, enjoy them in abundance. Try some new varieties, too.

Nuts and Seeds Try to get an ounce a day (a handful of nuts or two tablespoons of nut butter).

Vegetables Go crazy! Seriously, it's hard to get in seven to nine servings. Lean heavily on greens (raw or cooked), and eat colorful vegetables at every opportunity (golden peppers, red beets, purple potatoes, etc.) Consider a cup of greens or half a cup of other veggies to be a serving.

Whole Grains A good target is approximately a cup of grains or whole-grain pasta, or a generous slice of whole-grain bread. Avoid white flour as much as possible. Enjoy fermented (sourdough) breads and sprouted-grain breads whenever you can.

Would You Rather?

Eating just one meal out each week translates to a two-pound weight gain every year. On the other hand, cooking at home is strongly linked with longevity.

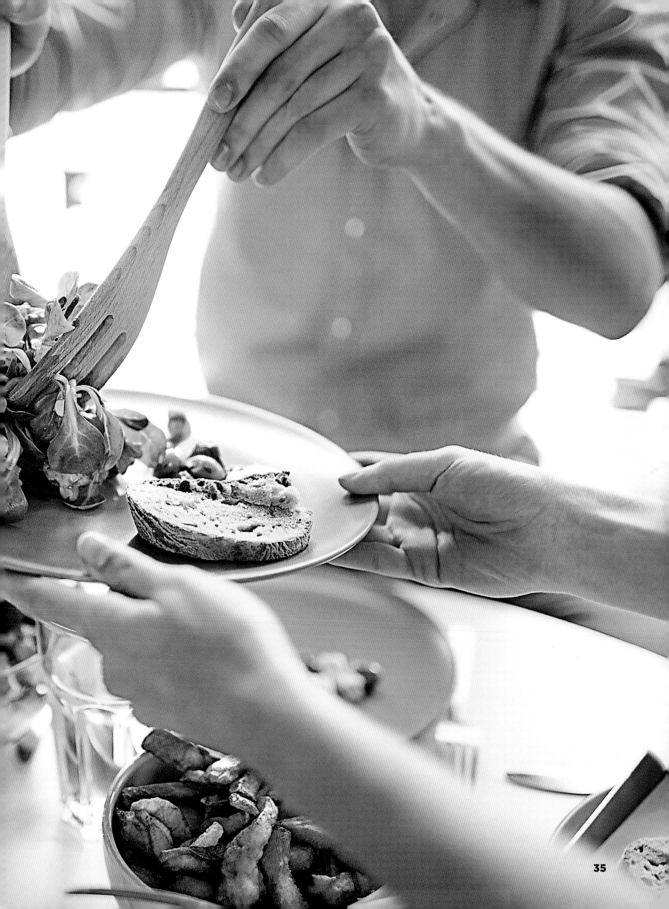

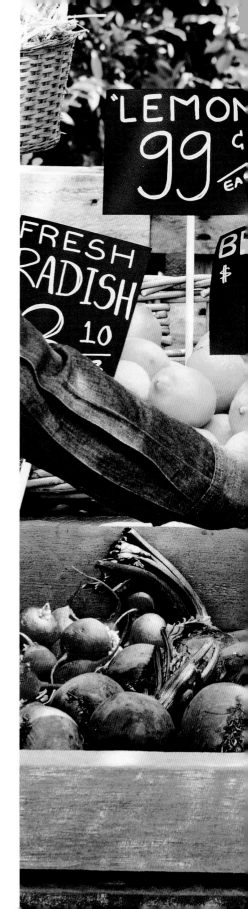

Shopping Tips for Affordable Goodness

You might think that buying healthier foods is a sure way to bust your budget. Think again! Fresh, high-quality nutrition doesn't have to be expensive. Follow these smart-shopping guidelines from Los Angeles nutritionist Lisa DeFazio, MS, RN, for ways to eat well that are gentle on your wallet.

Shop Local

When you get produce from a local stand, you save because "there are fewer hands involved," says DeFazio. "The farmer doesn't have to share his profits with the packer, the transporter, the corporation and store employees the way supermarkets do." Also, when you know the source, you can ask the seller directly about their farming practices and use of pesticides.

Time Your Purchases

Farmers work hard to come to market "first" or "last" with a certain crop because they can then charge more. "But if you wait until everyone at a market has a certain product—say tomatoes, or corn—the price will drop," explains DeFazio. Shopping at peak season is especially cost-efficient when you buy in bulk for canning or freezing.

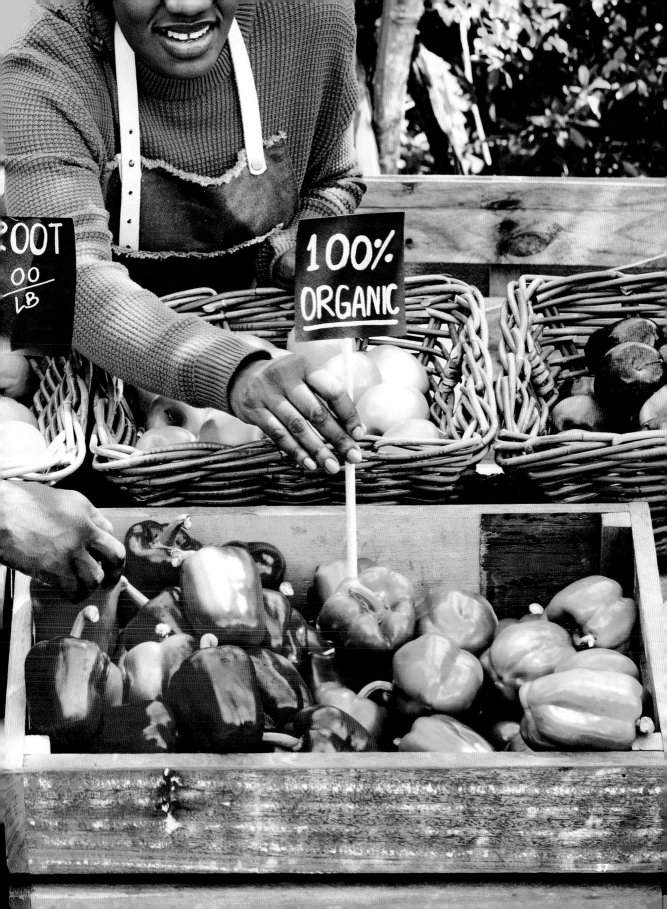

Become a Fan of Frozen

Don't go on a guilt trip if you can't make it to a farmer's market. Frozen produce is generally picked and preserved at peak ripeness, so it doesn't lose its potency during long-distance shipping. "Fruits and vegetables are often washed, blanched, frozen and packaged within a few hours of being harvested," says DeFazio. "I use frozen all the time!"

Grow Your Own

Of course, not everyone has a garden plot, but even if you have a sunny window or porch, you can cultivate herbs or a potted cherry-tomato plant. Over the course of the summer, you'll more than save what you spent on growing them yourself.

Go for Seconds

Markets often greatly discount imperfect produce, or "seconds." Sure, you might have to cut off a few brown spots, but your fruits and veggies will taste fine. And if you're just going to throw them in a skillet or blender, who cares what they look like?

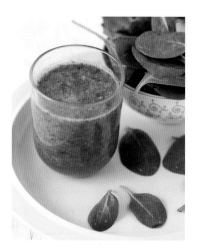

How to Keep Food Fresher, Longer

According to *Money* magazine, the average household tosses out nearly 15 percent of the food they buy because it's gone bad. That's a lot of wasted money over the course of a year! Here are some tips on how to keep your food edible.

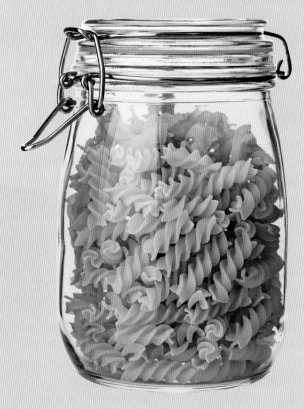

1 Wash berries with vinegar and water to keep them from getting moldy.

2 Transfer dry foods, such as pasta and cereal, into airtight containers when you bring them home.

3 Freeze flour for 48 hours—that will kill any insects that have snuck into the bag. Then transfer it to sealed containers.

4 Keep mushrooms in a paper bag. It absorbs moisture so they don't get slimy.

5 Remove celery from the plastic bag and wrap in foil for longer-lasting stalks that will stay crisp.

6 Stand asparagus on its cut end, in a shallow glass of water, in the fridge to keep it crisp.

Opt for organic as often as you can if you eat the skin of a fruit or veggie.

When to Buy Organic

For these three food groups, organic really matters.

FRUITS AND VEGETABLES
Nonorganic is OK for thick-skinned produce that you peel, but go organic for those on the "dirty dozen" list: strawberries, spinach, apples, grapes, peaches, cherries, pears, tomatoes, celery, nectarines, potatoes and peppers.

MEAT
The most important protein to buy organic may be beef. "Research suggests a strong connection between cancer in humans and hormones given to cattle," says DeFazio.

MILK
Yes, organic milk may cost twice as much, but considering how many hormones and antibiotics nonorganic dairy may contain, it's really worth the extra bucks for your family's peace of mind.

Smart Swaps

Clean up your grocery cart (and drop pounds!) with these satisfying and healthier substitutes.

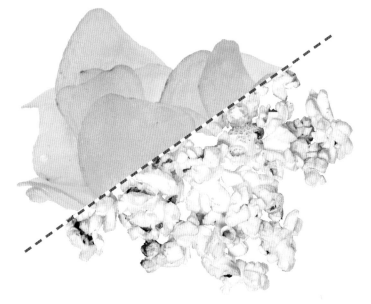

IF YOU LOVE SALTY/CRUNCHY FOODS...

Chips and crackers can have a place in a healthy diet—if you choose low-sodium, baked or homemade varieties. But if you're prone to overdoing it with stress-induced crunch cravings, try these alternatives.

SWAP

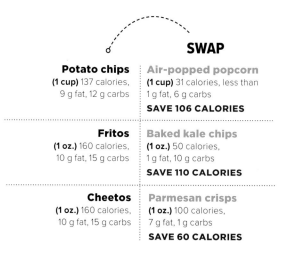

Potato chips (1 cup) 137 calories, 9 g fat, 12 g carbs	**Air-popped popcorn** (1 cup) 31 calories, less than 1 g fat, 6 g carbs **SAVE 106 CALORIES**
Fritos (1 oz.) 160 calories, 10 g fat, 15 g carbs	**Baked kale chips** (1 oz.) 50 calories, 1 g fat, 10 g carbs **SAVE 110 CALORIES**
Cheetos (1 oz.) 160 calories, 10 g fat, 15 g carbs	**Parmesan crisps** (1 oz.) 100 calories, 7 g fat, 1 g carbs **SAVE 60 CALORIES**

IF YOU CRAVE STARCHY CARBS...

For many of us, the thought of giving up bread and pasta is more than we can bear. But too many processed carbs (hello, mac and cheese!) are a slippery slope toward blood sugar problems—and worse. Exchange those for complex carbs, which have more fiber and less starch, for a comforting alternative.

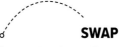

SWAP

Rice	**Riced cauliflower**
(1 cup) 206 calories, 45 g carbs, less than 1 g fat	**(1 cup)** 25 calories, 5 g carbs, less than 1 g fat
	SAVE 40 G CARBS
Pasta	**Zucchini noodles**
(1 cup, cooked) 220 calories, 43 g carbs, 1 g fat	**(1 cup)** 20 calories, 4 g carbs, less than 1 g fat
	SAVE 39 G CARBS
Granola	**Oatmeal**
(1 cup) 404 calories, 71 g carbs, 11 g fat	**(1 cup)** 150 calories, 26 g carbs, 2 g fat
	SAVE 45 G CARBS

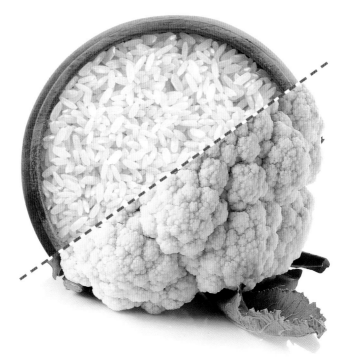

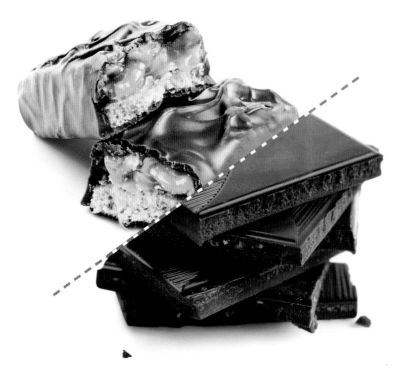

IF YOU HAVE A SWEET TOOTH...

Is it hard to feel satisfied without a little sweetness in your life? It doesn't hurt to indulge—and crush those sugar cravings. Just choose natural sweets rather than those with added sugar.

SWAP

Snickers bar **(1 small bar)** 215 calories, 20 g sugar, 11 g fat	**80 percent cocoa dark chocolate** **(1 oz.)** 170 calories, 7 g sugar, 12 g fat **SAVE 13 G SUGAR**
Ice cream **(1 cup)** 274 calories, 28 g sugar, 14 g fat	**Frozen banana** **(1 banana)** 105 calories, 14 g sugar, less than 1 g fat **SAVE 14 G SUGAR**
Chocolate pudding **(4 oz.)** 160 calories, 19 g sugar, 5 g fat	**Chia pudding** **(4 oz.)** 100 calories, 6 g sugar, 4 g fat **SAVE 13 G SUGAR**

IF YOU'RE A MEAT LOVER...

There's no need to give up meat in order to
lead a healthy lifestyle. But it does pay to limit
saturated fats and processed meats,
which are associated with certain cancer risks.
To get that umami flavor with less of the bad stuff,
go with leaner meats and vegetable stand-ins.

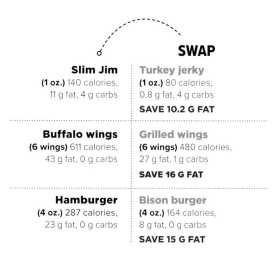

SWAP

Slim Jim **(1 oz.)** 140 calories, 11 g fat, 4 g carbs	**Turkey jerky** **(1 oz.)** 80 calories, 0.8 g fat, 4 g carbs **SAVE 10.2 G FAT**
Buffalo wings **(6 wings)** 611 calories, 43 g fat, 0 g carbs	**Grilled wings** **(6 wings)** 480 calories, 27 g fat, 1 g carbs **SAVE 16 G FAT**
Hamburger **(4 oz.)** 287 calories, 23 g fat, 0 g carbs	**Bison burger** **(4 oz.)** 164 calories, 8 g fat, 0 g carbs **SAVE 15 G FAT**

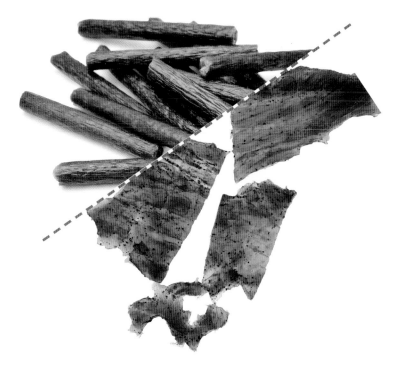

Sneaky Nutrient Boosts

Go nuts with these clever ideas for getting more of the best ingredients into every meal.

The easiest way to develop awareness of food choices is to stop and think before you prepare food: How can I make this more super? For the same quantity, could I get more power packed in? Is there a way to transform this choice into something that gives me energy instead of taking it away? Would it be possible to make this particular dish both tastier *and* more nourishing?

Eating well does not have to be about deprivation. There may be something beneficial you can add or swap. Think about ways you can replace one ingredient of little nutritive value with a better choice that satisfies the same craving or culinary purpose. What about adding one new superfood to your shopping cart with each trip to the grocery store? Or trying one superfood trick each day? How about this: Just add superfoods to your life, because they taste great and make you feel good!

Use the tips on the following pages as a launchpad to optimal health. And if you're worried about gaining weight by adding to your diet, consider this: Superfoods are packed with nutrition to fuel both brain and body. Start filling up your tank with more nutritious food and you may soon find your interest in foods that don't make you feel good waning. Eventually you'll be tucking tiny tastes of superfoods into everything: casseroles, hamburgers, tacos, sandwiches, frittatas, smoothies, soups, salads and stir-fries...Go crazy!

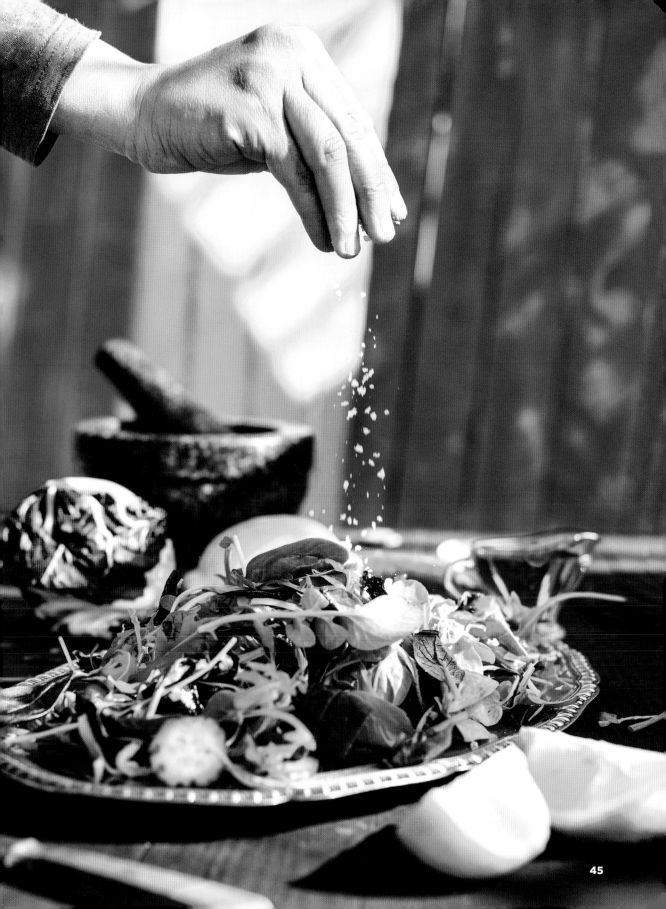

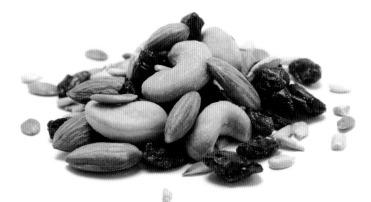

Sprinkle

- Add berries to every bowl of cereal and oatmeal.
- Add toasted nuts and seeds to both sweet and savory dishes.
- Garnish liberally with fresh herbs, sprouts and microgreens.
- Top roasted meats with sautéed mushrooms.
- Try plopping an anchovy or sardine on an otherwise plain green salad. You might be surprised!

Stir

- Add generous quantities of chopped, fresh herbs to beans, rice, polenta and scrambled eggs.
- Fold a tablespoon or two of ground flaxseed into batters and doughs.
- Include toasted nuts and seeds in egg salad and tuna salad mixtures, and in bread doughs.
- Spike mayo and mustard with garlic, herbs, lemon zest and pesto.

Fruitify

- Try to eat a different fruit every day.
- Reach first for fruit whenever you crave something sweet.
- Smash soft fruits, like bananas and peaches, into pancake batter.
- Put some fresh fruit on top when you enjoy dessert.

Vegify

- Try to eat a new vegetable every week.
- Include raw or cooked greens in every meal.
- Sauté garlic and veggies in olive oil before scrambling your eggs.
- Mix cooked vegetables into rice and grain sides.
- Add veggies whenever you make a filling, such as for enchiladas.
- Use avocado, hummus, miso and pesto as sandwich spreads instead of mayo.
- Use vegetable broth in place of water for cooking grains, beans, pasta, etc.

Tastify

- Use herbs and spices with abandon. Go for broke!
- Experiment with new flavors from the wide world of herbs and spices as often as possible.
- Add a small amount of a probiotic fermented item to almost all meals: sauerkraut, kimchi and pickles on the side, yogurt or miso stirred in, fermented soy sauce to season, and a good ale or wine to wash it all down.
- If a dish's flavor could use some brightening, try a little lemon or vinegar.

Dust

- Garnish eggs, popcorn and salads with savory nutritional yeast.
- Dust raw cacao powder onto yogurt and oatmeal, or sprinkle on a banana.
- Crumble roasted seaweed onto meat, fish, eggs, vegetables and mushrooms.

Drizzle

- Use a healthy oil (avocado, coconut, olive or walnut) to garnish cooked vegetables, salads and soups.
- Spoon plain yogurt onto chili, curries and stews.
- Spritz lemon or lime over chicken, fish and vegetables— and into a glass of water.

Hide

- Fold minced veggies into burgers, meatballs and meatloaf.
- Toss hearty greens into soups just before serving.
- Add a small handful of greens to all your frozen-fruit smoothies.
- Mix bitter greens, such as arugula, dandelion, endive and radicchio, with milder ones.
- Whisk roasted eggplant into dips and soups.
- Sub raw cacao powder for cocoa powder in chocolate recipes.

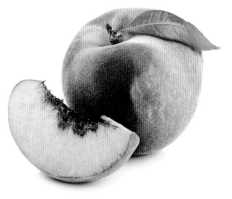

Swap This...for That

Try these super substitutions to up the nutrient ante one ingredient at a time.

FRESH WHOLE-WHEAT OR NUT FLOUR...
for white flour

GREEN TEA WITH STEVIA...
for soda

MASHED CAULIFLOWER...
for mashed potatoes

RICED CAULIFLOWER, BROWN RICE OR QUINOA...
for white rice

DRIED BERRIES...
for raisins in cereal and baked goods

SPROUTS...
for lettuce on sandwiches, burgers and tacos

COCONUT SUGAR, DATES, LUCUMA POWDER, MESQUITE FLOUR, YACÓN SYRUP OR STEVIA...
for refined white sugar

WHOLE FRUITS...
for fruit juices

DARK CHOCOLATE OR NUT BUTTER...
for high-sugar treats

EGGS IN THE MORNING...
for sugary cereals and pastries

SPAGHETTI SQUASH OR JULIENNED VEGETABLES...
for white-flour noodles

IN-SEASON PRODUCE...
for off-season produce

GRASS-FED MEAT, EGGS AND DAIRY...
for factory-farmed animal products

Nutrition Myths— Busted!

For most of us, it's time to rethink some long-held beliefs about our diets. Separating fact from fiction can help speed the process to a healthier you—and get you where you want to be.

Indulge in naturally low-cal berries!

Myth No. 1

All calories are created equal

We've all heard that the secret to weight loss is simple: Eat fewer calories and exercise more. But recent research shows the trick is to spend your caloric budget wisely. To get more for your calories, experts suggest, it's important to choose nutrient-dense foods, which, according to the National Institutes of Health and the U.S. Department of Health & Human Services, are foods that provide a high amount of nutrients but have relatively few calories. So for example, a small order of french fries contains 250 calories but very few nutrients. For the same number of calories, you could be eating heaps of fresh fruits and vegetables—10 cups of spinach, 1½ cups of strawberries and a small apple—which will flood the body with vitamins and minerals that will energize you and curb your hunger for hours.

TOP NUTRIENT-DENSE FOODS

Salmon

Seaweed

Kale, collard and dandelion greens

Blueberries

Shellfish

Spinach, arugula and watercress

Broccoli and cauliflower

Egg yolks

Nutrient-dense
superfood salmon
provides high
levels of protein
for relatively
few calories.

49

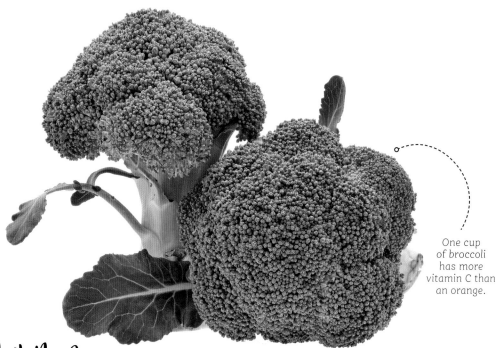

One cup
of broccoli
has more
vitamin C than
an orange.

Myth No. 2

Meat is king

Traditionally, we built meals around the almighty meat dish. But a growing body of research shows that we need less animal-based protein than previously believed—and more doctors are warning patients to eat less meat. "Remember that vegetables, beans and seeds are high in protein, so there is no essential need to have animal products at every meal," advises Joel Fuhrman, MD, author of *The New York Times* best seller *Eat to Live*. "In fact, broccoli has about the same amount of protein as steak."

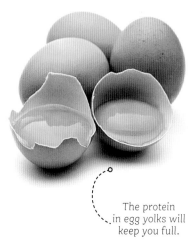

The protein
in egg yolks will
keep you full.

Myth No. 3

Fat makes you fat

One of the biggest obstacles to a healthier diet arose in the 1990s, with the denunciation of all fats and the rise of fat-free foods. Now those old theories are being punctured on a regular basis. A 2014 study published in the journal *Diabetes* found that unsaturated ("good") fat can help reduce abdominal fat while actually improving insulin production. Granted, we still need to limit saturated fats, like the kind found in processed baked goods and red meat. Those bad fats can juice up certain genes that increase the storage of fat in the belly, the *Diabetes* study said. On the other hand, healthy, unsaturated fats found in plants, oily fish and eggs can help to lower bad cholesterol, steady the blood sugar and aid in the absorption of other essential nutrients.

BAD FATS (SATURATED)	GOOD FATS (UNSATURATED)
Red meat	Avocado
Whole-fat dairy	Oily fish
Processed meat	Dark chocolate
Trans fat	Whole eggs
Partially hydrogenated oil	Nuts and seeds
Lard	Extra-virgin olive oil

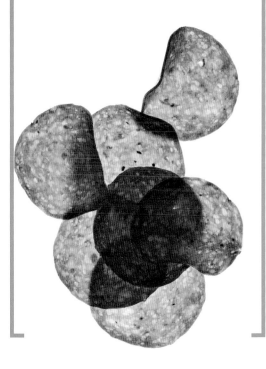

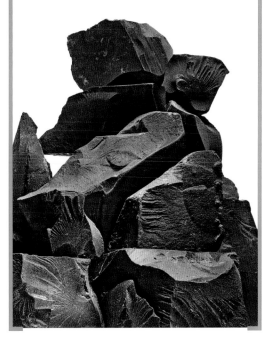

Myth No. 4

All carbs are evil

Carbohydrates are the devil in the minds of most dieters. But the truth is: Our bodies run on carbs. Researchers have proven time and again that a low-carb diet can make you feel tired, angry, depressed—even dizzy. So it's important to understand that, like fats, carbs come in different varieties: "good" (complex carbs) and "bad" (simple carbs).

The difference is in how quickly the sugar (which is essentially what carbohydrates are) is digested. Simple carbs, which include sugar-sweetened beverages, pastries, white bread, white pasta, white rice and many fruit juices, are low in fiber and are digested rapidly. This can cause drastic swings in blood sugar levels, leaving you hungry again in an hour. The result? Overeating.

On the other hand, complex carbs, which include vegetables, fruit, legumes, potatoes and whole grains, contain natural dietary fiber that helps curb hunger, and healthy plant compounds that rev up energy and lower your risk of chronic diseases. So go ahead and enjoy a little good starch!

Layer up! Add whole grains and fruit to Greek yogurt to burn belly fat and feel full for hours.

"Health Foods" That Aren't So Healthy

Watch out for these sneaky impostors!

By now, we know fat-free doesn't necessarily equal waist-friendly and that many gluten-free foods are packed with more calories than the foods they replace. But it's easy to get lulled into believing that an afternoon power bar or a post-dinner fro-yo is actually good for us. The truth is, many so-called healthy foods are anything but! Even people who are savvy about nutrition can get fooled by confusing labels and clever marketing. Stay on your toes with these tips from nutritionist Wendy Bazilian, DrPH, RDN, and author of *Eat Clean, Stay Lean: The Diet.*

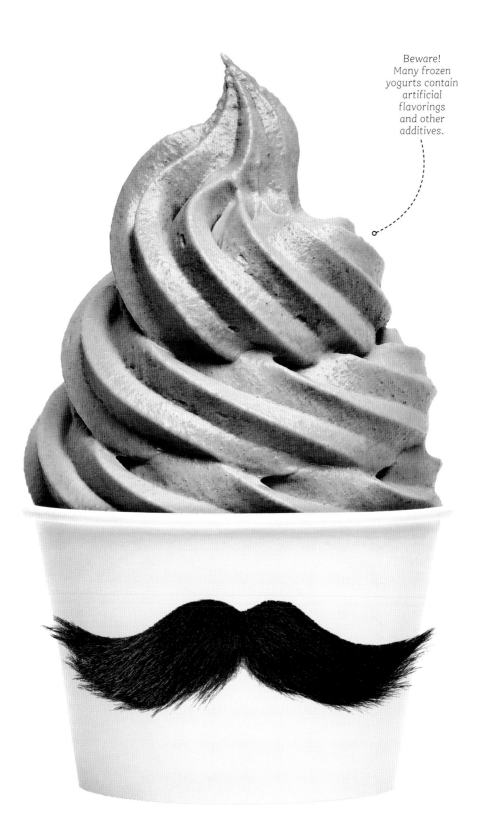

Beware! Many frozen yogurts contain artificial flavorings and other additives.

Frozen Yogurt

It sounds so virtuous. After all, yogurt is a nutritious source of calcium and protein and even offers probiotics to make our gut happy. But "if we're talking typical 'frozen yogurts,' the game changes," cautions Bazilian. "Most have 25 grams or more of sugar in only one-half cup—and that's without toppings!" You may be better off with a scoop of regular ice cream, Bazilian adds.

Energy Bars

They're super convenient and can be a great way to curb hunger. But many power bars are more like candy bars in "healthy" wrappings, with enough calories to equal an entire meal. "It's essential to look at the ingredients list," says Bazilian. "Some bars include artificial sweeteners, high-fructose corn syrup and high amounts of added sugars." Look for 10 or fewer ingredients and under 10 grams of sugar. Also, try for protein that comes from nuts, egg whites or pea protein, rather than soy protein isolate.

Multigrain (and Wheat) Bread

Multigrain sure sounds nutritious. We hear nearly every day the importance of whole grains, so having many of them must be good, right? "Technically, yes," says Bazilian. "But 'multigrain' does not always mean whole-grain. Typically, it just means 'many processed grains' combined in a single product." Wheat bread can be similar. If it doesn't say "whole wheat," it is simply made from a refined, enriched flour. "Check the ingredients list and look for the word 'whole,'" she adds. "It should be first on the list."

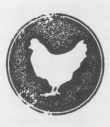 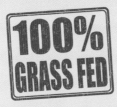

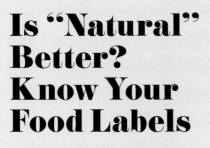

Is "Natural" Better? Know Your Food Labels

Trying to decipher labels when you're rushing to shop can be confusing at best. Use this glossary to make better choices in a snap.

NON-GMO
While "non-GMO" (genetically modified organisms) labels appear on many foods, the Non-GMO Project, a nonprofit organization, awards the most trustworthy products with its green Non-GMO Project label. These are certified by the organization, which ensures the foods are in no way genetically engineered. Check out the free Non-GMO Project shopping-guide app, which scans bar codes and searches the current list of products that have been verified.

USDA CERTIFIED ORGANIC
The USDA has strict production and labeling requirements for its organic labels. If a product claims to be USDA certified organic,

Veggie Chips

We know we need to eat more veggies, so it's easy to fall hook, line and sinker for these shrewdly named snacks. But be warned: "Most veggie chips are made with vegetable powder and are deep-fried, like potato chips—but without the benefit of real vegetables," says Bazilian. Some kale chips can offer good nutrition, she adds, and some freeze-dried veggies are actually made from the food they resemble. Look at the ingredients to be sure.

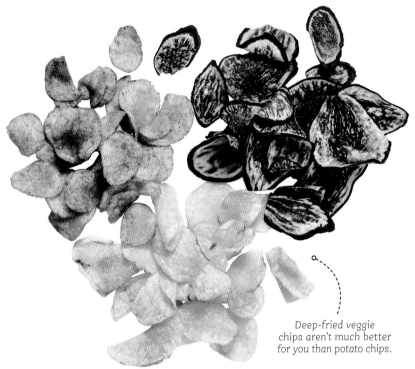

Deep-fried veggie chips aren't much better for you than potato chips.

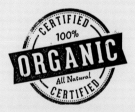

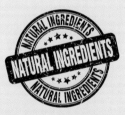

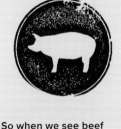

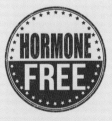

95 percent of the ingredients must have been grown or processed without synthetic fertilizers or pesticides. Animal products must not have received antibiotics of any type. In addition, organic foods cannot be genetically engineered or irradiated.

NATURAL
According to the USDA, "natural" means the product contains no artificial ingredients or added color and is only minimally processed. However, the food may contain antibiotics, growth hormones and other chemicals, which make the "natural" label all but worthless to anyone looking to avoid those additives.

HORMONE-FREE
Hormones naturally occur in all animals. So when we see beef or lamb that is labeled "Raised without hormones," this actually means that no *added* hormones were given and that the animals were raised in verified programs that are monitored by the USDA. As for pork and poultry, FDA regulations now prohibit any use of hormones in these products, so "hormone-free" is implicit.

GRASS-FED OR PASTURE-RAISED
"Grass-fed" is a certified USDA label that means an animal's primary source of food comes from grass or forage, not from grains. "Pasture-raised" means the animals spent at least some time in pasture, feeding on grass or forage—but may have been fed some grains.

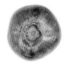

Foods That Help You Heal

From reducing inflammation to strengthening the immune system, foods are crucial to how our bodies react to stress and illness.

The ancient Greek physician Hippocrates is credited with the phrase, "Let food be thy medicine and medicine be thy food." Centuries later, we understand more than ever the close connection between food and pharmacology. Advances in nutrition science make it increasingly possible to pinpoint nutrients for their unique healing properties and to better understand the link between diet and disease. Consider these examples of the ways food can be medicine, and medicine can be food.

Note: Natural remedies are not meant as replacements for treatment by a medical professional. Never discontinue prescribed medications without first consulting your doctor.

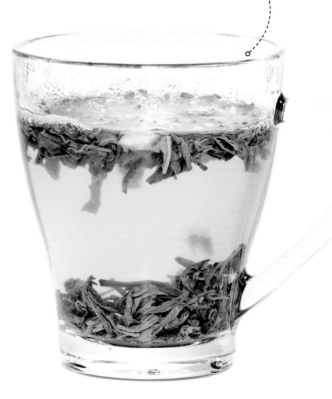

Drinking green tea speeds weight loss and burns belly fat, multiple studies show.

DETOX YOUR LIVER

The liver has been compared to a vacuum cleaner: It sucks up the dirt in our systems—an essential process for staying alive. With 25 percent of Americans now affected by fatty liver disease, caring for this hardworking organ should be high on your list. To support the liver, try kale and other dark, leafy vegetables. Research has shown that the glucosinolates in kale help regulate detoxification in our cells and aid in expelling harmful waste.

FEND OFF DIABETES

Type 2 diabetes is now nearly four times as common as all types of cancer combined. One of the best ways to fight it? Having two or more servings of brown rice per week is associated with a lower risk of developing type 2 diabetes, say researchers at the Harvard School of Public Health. On the other hand, they report, eating five or more servings of white rice per week can cause an increased risk. Fill up on other high-fiber foods as well, including beans and dark, leafy greens. Eating a diet high in fiber effectively lowers blood sugar levels, according to a review in the *Journal of the American Board of Family Medicine.* Women should aim for at least 25 grams of fiber per day and men for 30 grams per day.

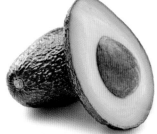

ELEVATE MOOD

Eat salmon, avocado and other foods rich in omega-3 fatty acids to improve your emotional well-being. Because our brains are about 60 percent fat, "the fatty acids from food help to insulate the nerve cells in the brain, allowing these cells to better communicate with one another," says Los Angeles nutritionist Lisa DeFazio, MS, RD. Insufficient levels of omega-3s are linked to depression, pessimism

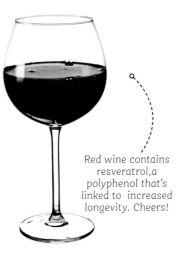

Red wine contains resveratrol, a polyphenol that's linked to increased longevity. Cheers!

and impulsivity. Meanwhile, researchers have found that depression rates are typically lowest in countries like Japan, where omega-3-rich fish is a diet staple. Avoid fast foods, many of which can cause or worsen depression, according to a 2012 study in the journal *Public Health Nutrition.*

PROTECT YOUR HEART

A heart-friendly diet can also be a fun one! You can sip red wine in moderation (resveratrol improves cardiovascular health) and eat blueberries with abandon. A 2015 study of women at Florida State University found that eating one cup of blueberries a day could significantly reduce blood pressure and stiff arteries. Meanwhile, eating a half-cup of nuts (not peanuts) each day has been shown to lower cholesterol and blood pressure without causing weight gain. Even better? "Eating one ounce of chocolate a day has been associated with a 45 percent lower risk of heart attack," says nutrition expert Jacob Teitelbaum, MD. "Compare this to just a 2 percent to 10 percent lower risk from cholesterol medications."

AMP METABOLISM

For a caffeine kick that will trim your waistline, start swilling green tea. Multiple studies show that people who drink green tea burn an extra 70 to 100 calories per day due to large amounts of the powerful catechin EGCG, which also helps prevent cancer. Another study found that metabolism sped up by 4 percent in 24 hours when people drank three to five cups of green tea per day. That's enough to lose seven pounds a year!

SUPERCHARGE YOUR IMMUNE SYSTEM

Red peppers are your go-to here, thanks to their intense concentration of vitamin C, a lack of which can make you more prone to getting sick. Just one medium-size bell pepper provides an astounding 253 percent DV of vitamin C. They're also jam-packed with phytochemicals and antioxidants, which power up the immune system and help turn on certain genetic switches to protect us from unfriendly invaders. It's essential to maintain daily intake of vitamin C, because your body doesn't produce or store it.

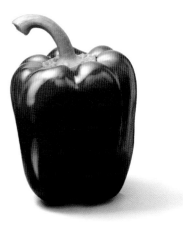

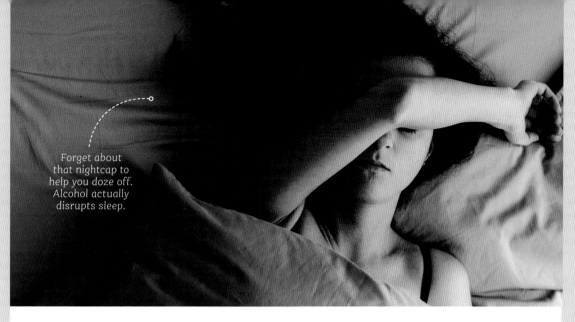

Forget about that nightcap to help you doze off. Alcohol actually disrupts sleep.

DO YOU NEED A DIET DO-OVER?

Many common ailments can be directly linked to food sensitivities.
If you're experiencing any of the conditions below, it may be time to tweak your menu.

CONDITION	SYMPTOMS	FOODS TO AVOID	FOODS TO EAT
HEARTBURN	Stomach pain, upper abdominal burning, chest pain, difficulty swallowing, chronic cough	Fried and fatty foods, tomatoes, citrus fruits, chocolate, garlic, onions, spicy foods, caffeine, mint	Ginger, nonacidic vegetables, oatmeal, noncitrus fruits, lean meats, egg whites, healthy fats
GLUTEN SENSITIVITY	Abdominal discomfort, brain fog, low energy, joint pain, headaches, skin problems, weight loss	Pasta, breads, pastries and other foods made with wheat or other grains containing gluten	Grain-free foods and wheat substitutes such as buckwheat, corn, millet, rice and quinoa
HEADACHES	Dull, aching head pain, tightness or pressure across the forehead or back of the neck	Diet drinks, soy sauce, MSG, alcohol, cured meats, gum, cheeses	Pumpkin seeds, potatoes (skin-on), cherries, cucumbers, chili peppers, complex carbs
INSOMNIA	Difficulty falling asleep, waking up in the night, waking up too early, not feeling rested after sleep	Caffeine, nightshade vegetables, alcohol, aged cheeses, cured meats, fermented foods, sugar, refined foods	Walnuts, bananas, tart cherry juice, basil
PREDIABETIC	Unexplained fatigue, excessive thirst, frequent urination, weight loss, blurred vision, cold hands and feet	Foods with added sugar, soda, pasta, white bread, white rice, fruit-flavored yogurt, sweetened breakfast cereals, dried fruits	Brown rice, greens, low-glycemic fruits and vegetables, steel-cut oats, lean meats, plain Greek yogurt, healthy fats
STRESS AND ANXIETY	Acne, headaches, rapid heartbeat, sweating, chronic pain, low energy, insomnia, depression, digestive distress	Refined sugar, caffeine, tofu, Chinese takeout, wheat bran, diet sodas	Bananas, spinach, olive oil, oats, salmon, strawberries, rooibos tea, dark chocolate, nuts

Superfoods, Super Mood

These foods improve energy, focus, mood, memory, sleep and more.

What we eat and drink profoundly affects how we feel—not just whether we are energetic or full, but also how we process emotions and memories, and whether we think clearly, sleep well, or suffer from anxiety and depression. The best advice for reducing your risk of various mental maladies is simply this: Eat tons of plants (vegetables, legumes, herbs, spices, fruit, nuts, seeds and whole grains). Get high-quality fats every day. It doesn't hurt to mix in some wild-caught fish and grass-fed animal proteins, too. Beyond these broad categories, certain specific foods also promote positive mental health by reducing irritability, relaxing the body and mind, increasing blood flow to the brain, creating new brain cells, and getting rid of toxins.

Brain-health and mood-disorder specialist Drew Ramsey, MD, has made "food as medicine" the focus of his clinical work. When he and his partners began prescribing nutrient-rich foods to patients, they started losing weight and feeling happier. Here are a few of the many examples of significant results from their Brain Food Clinic at Columbia University: A patient with panic attacks was cured by eating more seafood and having eggs for breakfast. Introducing seafood and lentils dramatically reduced one woman's severe anxiety. A teenager with irritability issues became calmer when he began to start the day with a smoothie made from fruit, yogurt and nuts. Dr. Ramsey thinks we all can benefit from fully fueling our brains—and it begins at the end of the fork.

BETTER SLEEP	CHILLING OUT	LASTING ENERGY	MEMORY AND FOCUS	LIFTING MOOD
Legumes, especially lentils	Chamomile tea	Grass-fed meat, eggs and dairy	Berries	Dark chocolate
Mushrooms	Dark chocolate	Green tea	Cinnamon	Fatty fish
Passionflower tea	Berries	Coffee	Grass-fed meat, eggs and dairy	Grass-fed meat, eggs and dairy
Chamomile tea	Hops (in tea or beer)	Legumes	Leafy greens	Quality fats
Root vegetables, ideally a few hours before bedtime	Lavender	Greens	Liver	Legumes
Warm milk (cows' milk or nut milk)	Lemon balm tea	Nuts and seeds	Nuts and seeds	Cooked spinach
	Mushrooms	Quality fats	Olives and olive oil	Mushrooms
	Black beans and soybeans	Fish and seafood	Sage	Olives and olive oil
	Wine (in moderation!)	Starchy, colorful vegetables	Seaweed	Rosemary
				Fermented foods

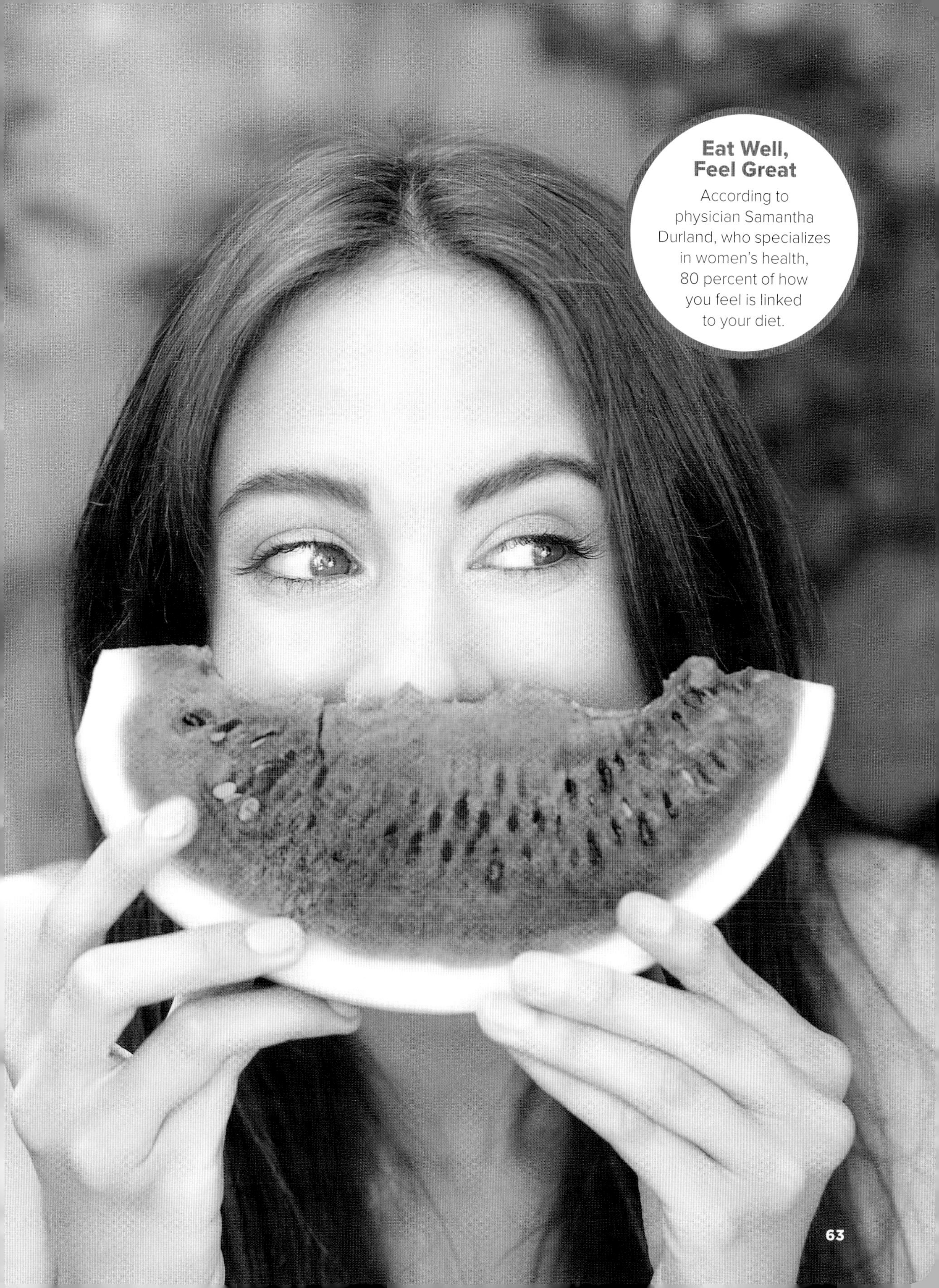

Eat Well, Feel Great

According to physician Samantha Durland, who specializes in women's health, 80 percent of how you feel is linked to your diet.

Fun Facts About Healthy Foods

Surprising foodie tidbits to tuck away for trivia night.

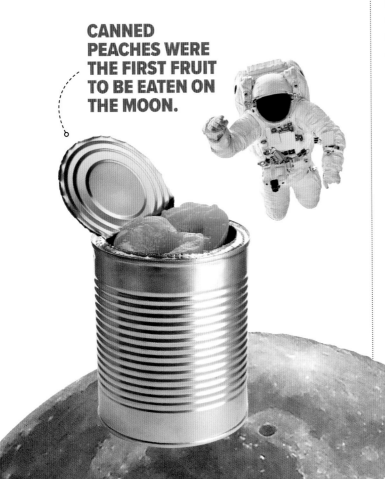

CANNED PEACHES WERE THE FIRST FRUIT TO BE EATEN ON THE MOON.

- You'll never need to throw out **honey**, because it never spoils. Scientists have found 3,000-year-old honey in Egyptian pyramids that was still perfectly edible! If it has crystallized, just microwave in short bursts, or put the jar in a bowl of hot water until it returns to normal consistency.

- According to the Koran, the Virgin Mary was fed **date-palm fruits** while in labor with the baby Jesus —to ease childbirth and give her strength.

- There are approximately 350 different pasta shapes around the world. Many Italians insist that the shape of the **pasta** affects the taste.

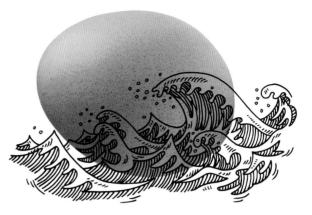

FRESH EGGS WILL SINK IN WATER, WHILE OLD EGGS TYPICALLY FLOAT— THAT'S A NEAT TRICK WHEN YOU'RE NOT SURE ABOUT THE CARTON YOU BOUGHT A FEW WEEKS AGO.

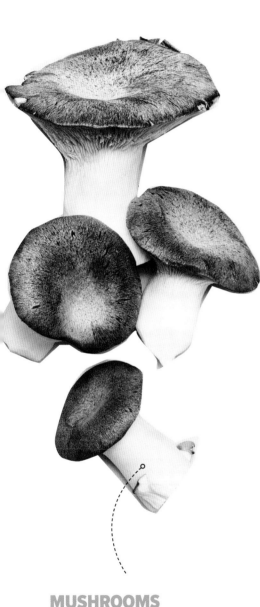

MUSHROOMS LOOK LIKE THEY'RE SOLID, BUT THEY ARE ACTUALLY 90 PERCENT WATER.

RAW LIMA BEANS CONTAIN THE LETHAL CHEMICAL COMPOUND CYANIDE. HOWEVER, THESE LITTLE BAD BOYS ARE SAFE TO EAT, SO LONG AS THEY ARE THOROUGHLY COOKED.

• If you're squeamish, skip this one. A number of European cheeses are illegal in the U.S. One of the most vile? **Casu marzu**, a Sardinian specialty, which is made with—wait for it—live maggots.

• **Egg yolks** are one of the few foods that naturally contain Vitamin D, the so-called sunshine vitamin.

• **Mushrooms** are impossible to overcook. Yes they might burn, but they will never become tough or bitter.

• **Chili peppers** are natural painkillers. The key is capsaicin, the chemical compound that gives peppers their heat. Capsaicin was first used to help ease the agony of shingles by applying it directly to the skin. It is now a common ingredient in creams and balms used to treat arthritis, fibromyalgia, back pain, shingles and postsurgical pain.

THE OYSTERS WE EAT ARE A
DIFFERENT SPECIES FROM THE ONES
THAT BEAR PEARLS. THE KIND THAT
ARE EATEN ARE CALLED OSTREIDS,
AND THE PEARL-PRODUCING OYSTERS
ARE CALLED PTEROIDA. SO FORGET
ABOUT FINDING A PEARL THE
NEXT TIME YOU ORDER OYSTERS.

• Are flamingos pink because they eat **shrimp**? Yes. The exotic birds get their vibrant coloring from eating brine shrimp, which are packed with beta-carotene—the same naturally occurring chemical that makes carrots orange. Likewise, if we humans eat a surfeit of carrots, our skin can turn orange.

• Thomas Jefferson was quite the culinary pioneer. He is credited with introducing **pasta** to the U.S., as well as **broccoli** and other vegetables that he encountered in France.

BEFORE THE 2012 KALE CRAZE HIT, PIZZA HUT WAS REPORTEDLY THE LARGEST CONSUMER OF KALE IN THE U.S.— THE RESTAURANT CHAIN USED IT AS GARNISH FOR ITS SALAD BARS.

• The Yubari King **cantaloupe** from Japan is the most expensive fruit in the world. A pair of the rare, sweet fruits fetched $27,295 at auction.

• A **lemon** contains more sugar than an extra-large **strawberry**.

WHEN EUROPEAN EXPLORERS FIRST SAW PINEAPPLES, THEY THOUGHT THEY LOOKED LIKE PINE CONES—WHICH IS HOW THE TROPICAL FRUIT GOT ITS NAME.

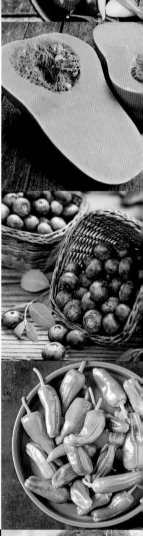

PART 2

A-Z

Superfoods

GUIDE

Nutrient- and energy-dense food comes in many satisfying forms. Try adding these ingredients to your diet to boost nourishment while bringing new flavors to the table.

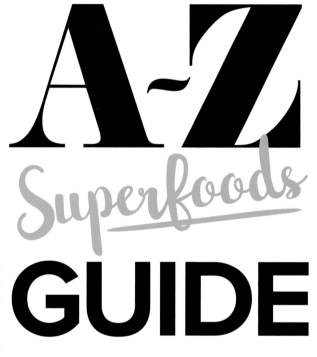

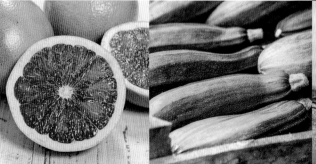

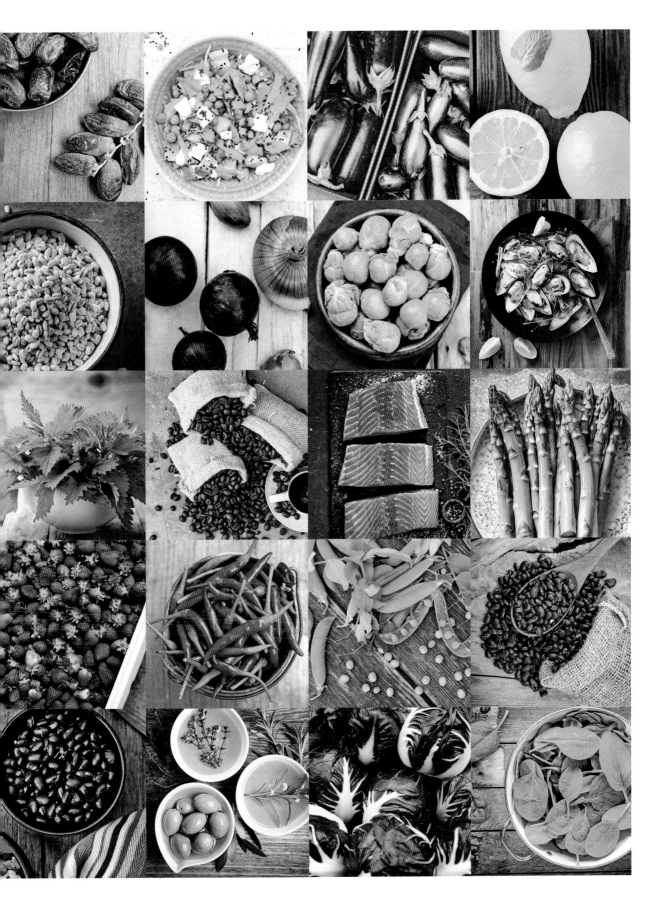

Açai Berry

It's worth getting to know this uncommon fruit for both its rich flavor and healthful properties.

The culinary and health potential of açai (pronounced ah-sah-ee) berries have many intrigued. First, there's the taste: These dark-purple berries of the açai palm, native to Central and South America, are often described as having a mix of berry and chocolate flavors. They also are unusually rich in antioxidants, more than most of the other berries found in grocery stores. Much research on these nutritious berries remains to be done, but some early studies look promising: Emerging research suggests that this berry may have a beneficial effect on both blood-sugar and cholesterol levels.

ALSO TRY Red **goji berries** are another antioxidant-rich berry packed with potential. These tart fruits are native to China, where they are used medicinally. Most often in the West, you'll find them dried. They add appealing crunch to whatever you toss them into.

SCIENCE SAYS

A 2016 article in the American Journal of Clinical Nutrition found that for a group of overweight men, consuming açai-based smoothies was associated with improvements in vascular function. These changes may lower the risk of a cardiovascular event.

How to Buy & Enjoy

• Açai berries are often sold as a frozen puree or pulp, which is easy to add to smoothies or thaw out for a breakfast bowl. • Açai also shows up in juice blends, but beware of added sugar when buying juice. • If you visit South America, enjoy them fresh! Açai berries can't be shipped to the United States because they go rancid shortly after being picked.

Artichoke

This versatile vegetable boasts berry-like antioxidant levels!

A Mediterranean staple, artichokes are often overlooked in North America (except in restaurant spinach dips). The part of the plant we eat is a huge flower bud full of beneficial compounds. In particular, artichokes are a good source of a type of antioxidant called polyphenols, which may help prevent many diseases. Artichokes are also high in fiber; important for digestive health; and a good source of vitamins C and K, folate, magnesium and manganese. According to Jo Robinson, who has researched nutrient levels in everyday foods for more than a decade, artichokes are one of the healthiest foods you can get from any grocery store. Fresh is great, but even canned artichokes are supremely nutritious; you'd have to eat 30 servings of carrots to get the same benefits!

ALSO TRY Other foods rich in polyphenol antioxidants that support the heart, brain and body include **berries**, **wine**, **coffee** and **tea**.

How to Buy & Enjoy

- Bitter compounds in artichokes are balanced by the richness of butter, mayo and creamy sauces. The classic French preparation is to fill the center of a boiled artichoke with hollandaise sauce. ● This hardworking vegetable wears many hats. Try artichokes boiled, stuffed, roasted, grilled and even chilled.
- Cooking an artichoke boosts antioxidant levels. ● Beware of pairing artichokes with wine—they can make some wines taste extra sweet. It's best to go with a bone-dry white wine, such as sauvignon blanc.

The dark-green outer part of the flesh is the most nutritious.

Avocado

Once a guilty pleasure, this gem is now recognized as a nutritional powerhouse.

For years, dieters avoided avocados for fear of fat and calories. But no more! Avocados are now considered a surprisingly healthy choice. They are a good source of potassium, folate and vitamins C and K. Avocados are also full of fiber, and the fat is mainly monounsaturated —which helps decrease levels of LDL, or "bad" cholesterol. They even help increase satiety (the feeling of fullness), which can aid in maintaining a healthy weight. Be sure to scrape all the nutrient-rich flesh out of the peels, especially the darker-green outer part.

ALSO TRY "Natural" or minimally processed versions of **almond, cashew, peanut** and other **nut butters** are good sources of plant-based fats as well as numerous vitamins and minerals.

How to Buy & Enjoy

● Consider avocados a superfood alternative to heavily processed condiments like margarine and mayo.
● Use semifirm avocados to cut slices and cubes to add to salads and tacos; choose softer avocados for guacamole and as a condiment. ● Mix up your morning routine by swapping out cereal for avocado on whole-grain toast sprinkled with salt. ● Avocado also increases creaminess in smoothies; its flavor hides behind sweet fruits and toasted nuts.

Barley

Heart-healthy barley
is full of whole-grain
goodness, great flavor
and chewy texture.

In North America, whole-grain barley
is more commonly used in animal feed
and beer—but it has a lot to offer as an
everyday food. In the Mediterranean,
barley is a staple grain, and has been
identified as the single food most
associated with living to be 100 years old.
Barley is full of soluble fiber, which helps
stabilize blood-sugar and cholesterol
levels. It also packs a boatload of
vitamins and minerals, which is especially
impressive in terms of daily values when
consumed as "hulled" barley.

ALSO TRY Consume a wide variety
of minimally processed whole grains
(less processing means more nutrients)—
especially **oats**, another source of soluble
fiber that is especially good for the heart.
An easy way to get more whole grains is
to eat **low-sugar**, **whole-grain cereals**
for breakfast.

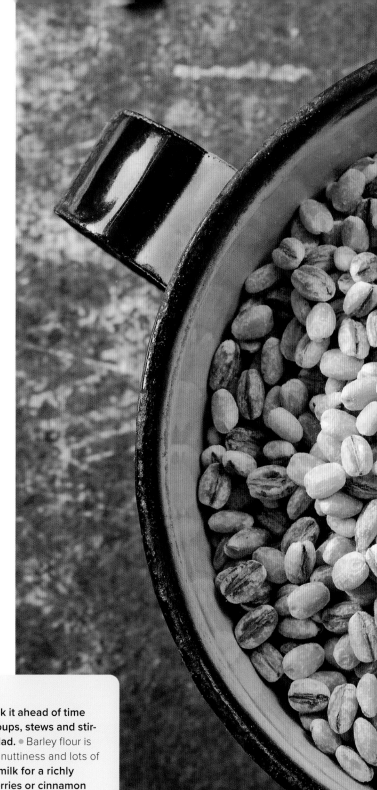

How to Buy & Enjoy

● **Barley is common in soups. You can cook it ahead of time
and refrigerate. Then add as needed to soups, stews and stir-
fries, or transform it into a whole-grain salad.** ● Barley flour is
wonderful in baked goods, adding a bit of nuttiness and lots of
moisture. ● **Cook barley in apple juice or milk for a richly
flavored hot cereal. Top with nuts and berries or cinnamon
and yogurt.** ● Although pearled barley (which has the outer
bran removed) has less fiber than hulled barley, it's still a good
source of fiber. Also look for hull-less versions.

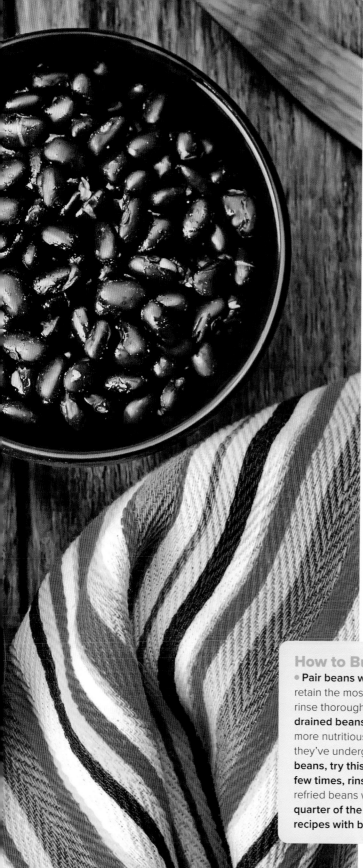

Black Bean

This kitchen staple is a great source of fiber and plant-based protein.

All beans are excellent sources of plant-based protein, and black beans in particular have much to offer. They are packed with antioxidants, including anthocyanins. These are the dark antioxidant pigments also found in red wine and red cabbage. Black beans are a good source of many of the most underconsumed nutrients, such as fiber, folate and magnesium. Combine them with rice, and you have an excellent source of complete protein—which makes this easy combo a favorite of vegetarians and people trying to consume less meat.

ALSO TRY In most recipes, you can substitute small **red beans** or **red kidney beans** for black beans; both varieties are super high in antioxidants.

How to Buy & Enjoy

● **Pair beans with rice for complete plant protein.** ● To retain the most nutrients in dry beans: Soak overnight, rinse thoroughly and cook in a pressure cooker. ● **Add drained beans to salads.** ● Canned beans are actually more nutritious, because of the high-heat production they've undergone. ● **If you have a hard time eating beans, try this: Pour off and refresh the soaking liquid a few times, rinsing thoroughly each time.** ● Try swapping refried beans with mashed black beans. ● **Replace one-quarter of the white flour in chocolate cake and brownie recipes with black-bean flour.**

Blueberry

Eat this berry because it's yummy—or because tons of nutrition research backs up its benefits.

Blueberries are native to North America, which makes it easier to find fresh and local varieties than some other superfood fruits. Both wild and cultivated blueberries are full of nutrients (especially the tiny and dark wild kinds). Blueberries contain dietary fiber as well as vitamins C and K, but what may be most interesting about blueberries is that they're packed with antioxidants. Specifically, they're high in anthocyanins, which may have benefits for heart health. Whatever the mechanism, studies have found that blueberries are associated with a number of health benefits, including improved insulin sensitivity and protection of mental function as well as lowered risk of heart disease.

ALSO TRY Several other dark berries—including **mulberries**, **maqui** and **strawberries**—are rich in anthocyanin pigments and may have similar health properties to blueberries (turn page for more).

How to Buy & Enjoy

- After harvest, blueberries will continue to develop aroma—but not sweetness. Whenever possible, try to eat them shortly after they've been picked. • Blueberries retain flavor, nutrients and shape quite well when frozen or baked. To store extra berries, freeze them in a single layer, not touching, on a sheet pan. When they are frozen solid, move them to a sealed container. • When baking with blueberries, be sure the baking soda is thoroughly incorporated throughout the batter, and try to use the least amount of baking soda possible. The alkalinity can turn the berries green. Adding an acid, such as lemon juice, also helps retain their color. • A small but interesting study found that blueberries may lose some antioxidant benefits when consumed with milk.

BLACKBERRIES
Wild blackberries have the most antioxidants—a good reason to go berry-picking!

STRAWBERRIES
Strawberries are fighters: They battle cataracts, headaches, wrinkles, inflammation and cancer.

CRANBERRIES
Antibacterial cranberries inhibit urinary tract infections, food-borne pathogens and the growth of cancer cells.

MORE BERRY POWER

The delicious fruits have a remarkable ability to reverse the ravages of time.

Rich in fiber, minerals and vitamins, berries are antioxidant powerhouses, helping to fight disease, slow the aging process and boost health. Enjoy them in abundance—alone as nature's candy, in pancakes and muffins, on yogurt or in smoothies. If it's not summertime, choose frozen berries, which are still supernutritious and packed with flavor.

GOLDENBERRIES
Low-sugar goldenberries, or husk cherries, strengthen immunity through their bioflavonoids.

BLUEBERRIES
Consume brain-boosting blueberries daily to dramatically slow the effect of aging on memory and motor skills.

AÇAI BERRIES
Eat fresh or frozen Brazilian açai berries for their cholesterol-lowering sterols and intense flavor.

RASPBERRIES
You'll get more fiber from raspberries than from a bran muffin.

CAMU CAMU BERRIES
Tropical camu camu berries have up to 60 times more vitamin C than an orange.

MAQUI BERRIES
Dark purple maqui boasts the most antiaging antioxidants of any fruit.

GOT MOLD?
Try this tip from *Cook's Illustrated* magazine to keep from throwing out fresh berries: Wash them in a 3:1 water-to-vinegar solution, then rinse, gently dry and refrigerate them in a towel-lined, partially open container.

MULBERRIES
Mulberries are one of the few food sources of the antiaging antioxidant resveratrol.

SEA BUCKTHORN
Orange sea buckthorn has an impressive ability to keep skin healthy and rejuvenated.

Coconut

This versatile fruit has a lot going for it—when used in moderation.

There's plenty of good stuff inside the coconut. The raw meat of this large nut contains dietary fiber and many vitamins and minerals—it's especially high in manganese. Coconut is also quite functional in cooking. If you're on a gluten-free or vegan diet, using coconut oil (a solid fat, like butter) or coconut flour in baked goods opens up a wide range of culinary possibilities. Include coconut with other whole foods in an overall balanced diet. Be sure not to let it replace all your heart-healthy olive oil, however!

ALSO TRY **Figs** and **dates** also have sweet culinary potential. Try them as substitutes for some of the sugar in your baked goods, adding lots of nutrients and fiber.

How to Buy & Enjoy

- When buying flaked and shredded coconut meat, look for unsweetened. It's naturally sweet already!
- Toasting coconut deepens nuttiness and changes the texture.
- Creamy coconut milk is a nutritious base in which you can cook everything from rice to chicken.
- Freeze coconut water in ice cube trays to use in drinks and smoothies.

SCIENCE SAYS

Experts argue over the pros and cons of coconut, especially its oil. The main issue is the saturated fat (which makes it solid). Research suggests the virgin oil behaves less like other saturated fats and actually raises HDL (good) cholesterol when consumed in moderation.

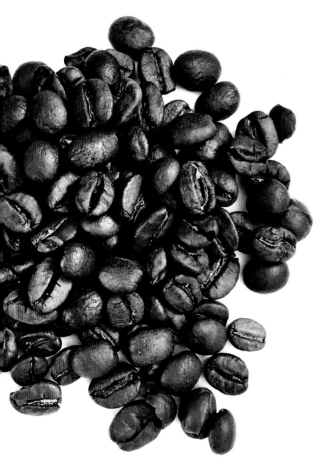

Coffee

The latest research on coffee continues to suggest numerous health benefits.

Few foods or beverages can boast as many potential health benefits as coffee. Studies suggest that it may help protect against heart disease, liver disease, Parkinson's disease, diabetes and some kinds of cancer, and that it can also combat depression and improve cognitive function. While many of these positive effects are associated with caffeine, some benefits may be due to the hundreds of other compounds in coffee. In fact, while less studied, even drinking decaf coffee appears to offer health benefits.

ALSO TRY Don't happen to like coffee? That's OK. You have options! Both **green tea** and **red wine** are high in polyphenols, and tons of studies have suggested health benefits for those beverages as well. Green tea may help protect against heart disease, liver disease and different cancers. The risks and benefits of red wine are more complicated, because it's not always clear how alcohol affects cancer risk. However, research suggests that moderate consumption of red wine may protect against heart disease. Not to be overlooked: There are also plenty of health benefits associated with drinking just plain **water**!

How to Buy & Enjoy

● **Hot or cold, coffee is beneficial—but note that these benefits have nothing to do with added sweeteners.** ● Keep coffee drinking to the early part of the day to avoid sleep disruption. Pregnant women also are advised to limit caffeine intake, especially during the first trimester. ● **Coffee can be used as a rich, acidic ingredient in baking recipes, such as chocolate cake.** ● For the freshest cup: Keep recently roasted, whole beans in the freezer to grind just before brewing.

SCIENCE SAYS

A 2017 review of the major research to date on coffee from the publication BMJ found that drinking moderate amounts of coffee reduced the risk for a number of health conditions, including cardiovascular disease, liver disease and several types of cancer.

Cheese

From soft and creamy to firm and flavorful, find your favorite variety.

Good news! Cheese can be as healthy as it is delicious. A 2015 Danish study debunked the traditional wisdom that saturated fats in dairy are bad for our hearts. In fact, it showed that eating cheese lowered bad cholesterol levels and cut the risk of heart disease. But before you go running for the comfort of a Camembert, be aware that no two types of cheese are exactly alike. While texture, moisture content, age and flavor all differ widely, so do their rankings on the health scale. The varieties below are considered the healthiest choices—but are still best enjoyed in moderation.

GRUYÈRE
Aged cheeses, like gruyère, are rich in butyrate, a fatty acid effective in warding off obesity and reducing the risk of type 2 diabetes.

PECORINO ROMANO
This hard, salty Italian staple made from sheep's milk has three to five times the conjugated linoleic acid (CLA) found in cow's cheese. CLA is helpful in reducing body fat, preserving muscle and improving bone health.

MOZZARELLA
The world is a happier place, thanks to this melty mouth-pleaser. Lucky for us, 1.5 ounces of this delicious treat has 333 milligrams of calcium—the highest of all types of cheese.

How to Buy & Enjoy
- To maintain moderation (one ounce per day of full-fat cheese), try shredding and sprinkling on sandwiches or salads rather than eating whole slices or chunks.
- Be sure to grate your own to avoid additives like cellulose (aka wood-chip powder).
- Look for flavor cues on the package—words like creamy, soft, tangy or robust, which indicate the taste profile.

PARMESAN
This aged ace is the protein champ of the cheese world, with a whopping 10 grams per ounce. (Most other cheeses contain an average of six to seven grams per ounce.)

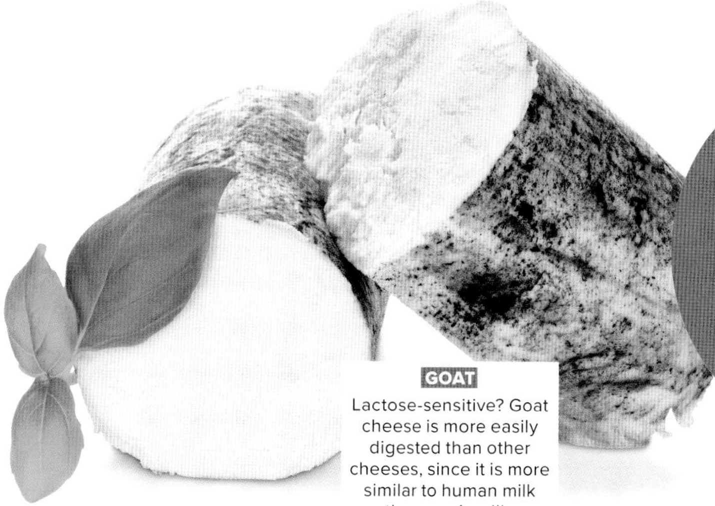

GOAT

Lactose-sensitive? Goat cheese is more easily digested than other cheeses, since it is more similar to human milk than cow's milk.

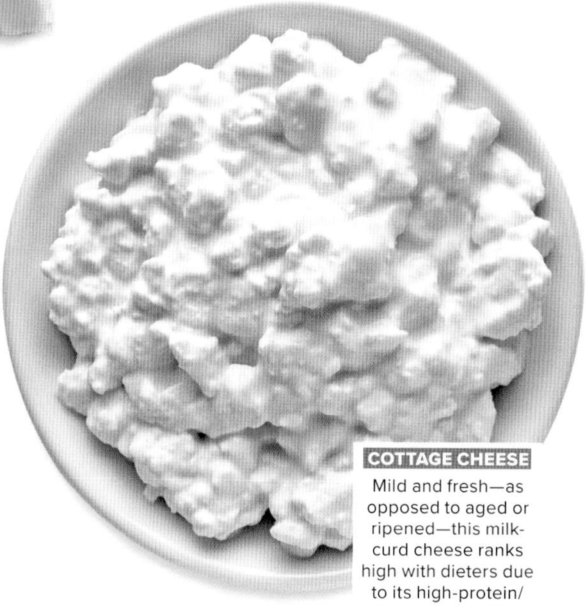

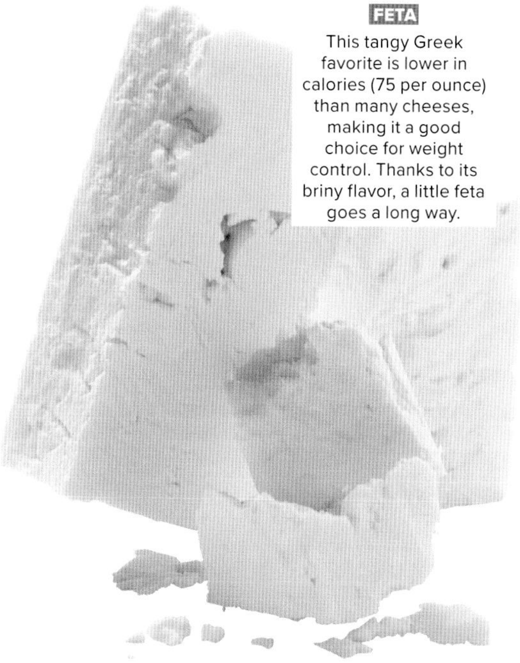

SCIENCE SAYS

These healthy cheeses are all outstanding sources of calcium, which protects against osteoporosis as well as cancer, diabetes and high blood pressure. They also pack plenty of protein, which steadies blood sugar levels, makes you feel full, and builds lean muscle.

FETA

This tangy Greek favorite is lower in calories (75 per ounce) than many cheeses, making it a good choice for weight control. Thanks to its briny flavor, a little feta goes a long way.

COTTAGE CHEESE

Mild and fresh—as opposed to aged or ripened—this milk-curd cheese ranks high with dieters due to its high-protein/low-calorie ratio.

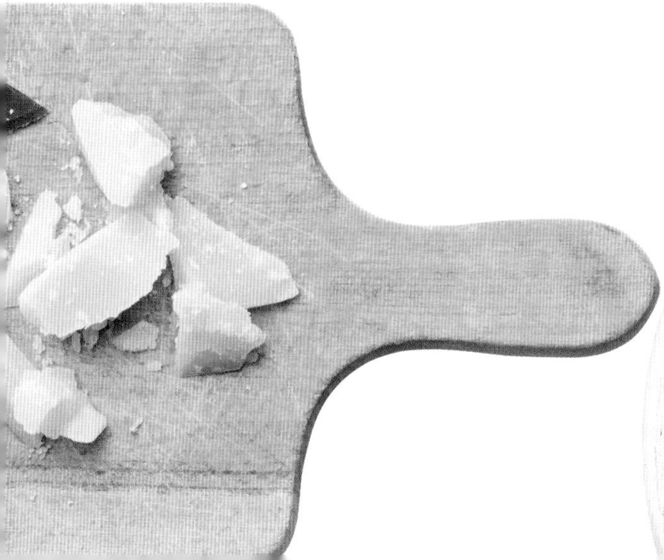

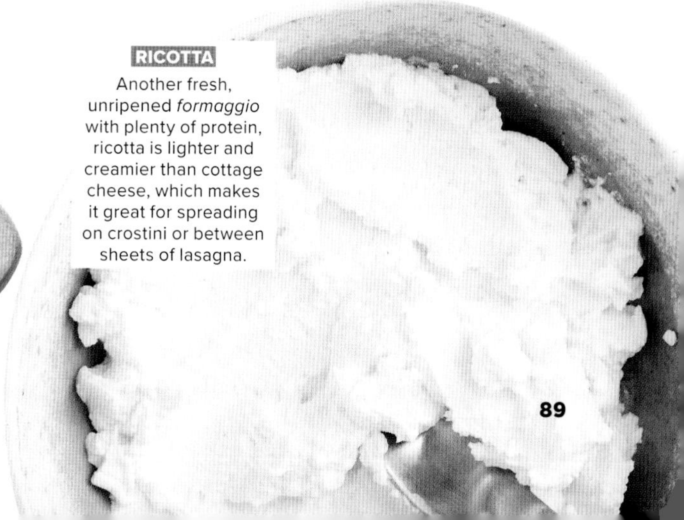

RICOTTA

Another fresh, unripened *formaggio* with plenty of protein, ricotta is lighter and creamier than cottage cheese, which makes it great for spreading on crostini or between sheets of lasagna.

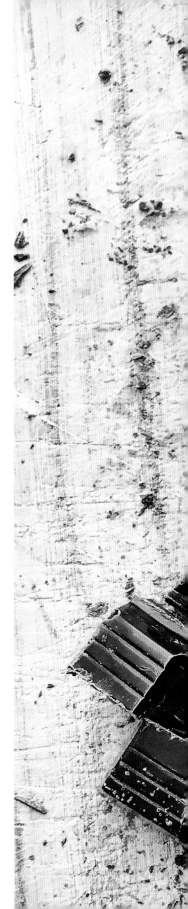

Dark Chocolate

Not too good to be true—the flavorful compounds in dark chocolate have serious health benefits.

For those who enjoy the rich taste of dark chocolate, you're in luck! The compounds that give dark chocolate its slightly bitter flavor are associated with numerous benefits for heart health, and they're found at much greater concentrations in dark chocolate than in milk chocolate. Research suggests flavanol-rich dark chocolate may have positive effects on insulin sensitivity, blood pressure and cholesterol levels as well. Chocolate is also a good source of two often underconsumed minerals: iron and magnesium. Most experts suggest chocolate be consumed in moderation, but an ounce or two per day of the good stuff can be pretty satisfying. Surprise benefit: Eating dark chocolate can increase satiety—decreasing feelings of hunger that lead to overeating. Chocolate also has been found to reduce cravings for something sweet.

ALSO TRY Like dark chocolate, **nuts** are relatively high in calories. But they're great for your heart, and they fill you up, so moderate intake may help you lose extra weight.

How to Buy & Enjoy

● **Store chocolate in a cool, dark, dry place to keep it for up to a couple of years.** ● Look for products with at least 70 percent cacao (or more). These contain the most flavanols. ● **Also look for products that have not been "Dutch processed," which reduces the health benefits.** ● When buying chocolate, pay attention to ingredients; avoid brands that contain excess refined sugars; additives, such as soybean oil; and emulsifiers, like soy lecithin.

SCIENCE SAYS
Polyphenols in dark chocolate, specifically flavanols, may have many beneficial effects. Looking at the difference between flavanol-rich dark chocolate and flavanol-free white chocolate, research suggests the dark version can improve both blood pressure and blood sugar.

SCIENCE SAYS

Dates are rich in fiber and antioxidants, which may improve digestive health. Some studies suggest that consuming dates may reduce the risk of colon cancer. For example, a 2015 study of 22 volunteers found that eating palm dates improved markers for colon health.

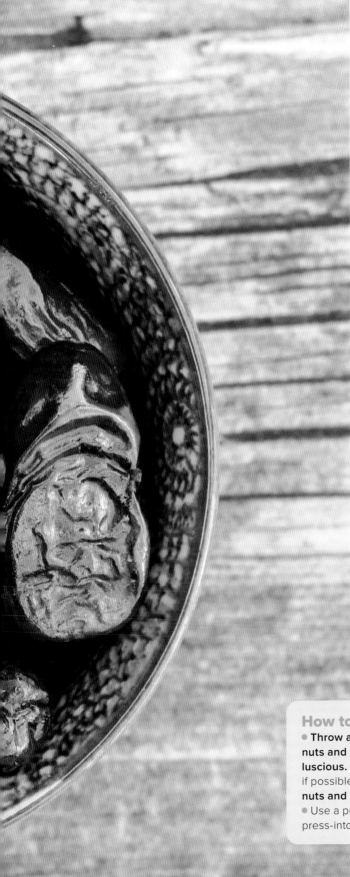

Date

This sugar alternative is loaded with essential vitamins and nutrients.

The fruit of the date palm tree is a staple crop in many parts of North Africa and West Asia. Dates are rich in fiber and polyphenol compounds. A single date contains small amounts of many nutrients, including potassium and magnesium. Because they contain a lot of natural sugar, dates aren't a food you want to eat immoderately. But they're an excellent natural sweetener and a pretty good substitute for refined sugar in many recipes.

ALSO TRY **Figs** and **coconuts** can be used in baking to add sweetness in conjunction with fiber and other nutrients.

How to Buy & Enjoy

● **Throw a couple of dates in a blender with fruits, nuts and milk to make smoothies sweeter and more luscious.** ● To retain fiber and nutrients, use whole dates, if possible. ● **Pureed dates are a good binder. Blend with nuts and seeds to make simple, flavorful energy bars.** ● Use a puree of dates and nuts or nut flours for delicious press-into-the-pan pie crusts.

How to Buy & Enjoy

• **Smaller eggplants will taste sweeter.** • The sourish, bitter flavor of eggplant becomes more mellow and complex via roasting and smoking. • **Depending on your recipe and the texture you desire in a finished eggplant dish, you may want to remove excess moisture ahead of time by salting the flesh and then patting it dry.** • Eggplants are best enjoyed fresh. To maintain flavor, color and nutrients, always store at room temperature rather than in the refrigerator.

Eggplant

For the greatest health benefits, be sure to eat that purple peel.

Eggplant is an important food in global cuisine, especially popular in Italy and elsewhere in the Mediterranean. This creamy-meaty vegetable is found in many vegetarian dishes. Cooks also enjoy its ability to absorb other flavors. High in fiber and low in calories, you can find tons of healthy recipes featuring eggplant, including many developed specifically for diabetics. However, because eggplant also absorbs fat easily, keep an eye on ingredient quantities. Otherwise, you may not notice how much salt, fat and spice the eggplant flesh is absorbing. You'll also want to leave the skin on to get the most antioxidants.

ALSO TRY Squash is another example of a high-fiber, low-calorie food with versatile uses in healthy recipes, because it can absorb a lot of flavor.

Fig

This delicious fruit is another sweet alternative to refined sugar.

Native to the Mediterranean and West Asia, these aromatic dewdrops are a treat when eaten fresh and are beloved wherever they grow. They're the food most frequently mentioned in the Bible. Dried figs are different but still delicious—and quite useful. They add natural sweetness to baked goods and are surprisingly high in fiber, largely from the many small seeds. Half a cup has more than seven grams of fiber! Figs also have lots of antioxidants, vitamins and minerals, including potassium, manganese and B vitamins.

ALSO TRY Most fruits are fiber-full, especially if they have tons of tiny seeds. **Blackberries** and **raspberries** have about eight grams per cup.

How to Buy & Enjoy
● **Many North Americans have never had fresh figs, but these perishable treats are worth seeking out for the delicate flavor.** ● Figs dry easily in a natural process that usually begins on the tree. Try the many diverse and differently colored versions. Some are sweeter, some are spicier, some are more caramel-like. ● **Blend figs into a paste with nuts and press the mixture into tins to make fiber-rich crusts for tarts and pies.** Sweet figs have enough richness to stand up to being paired with roasted meats and vegetables, and they also make wonderfully thick and syrupy fruit vinegars.

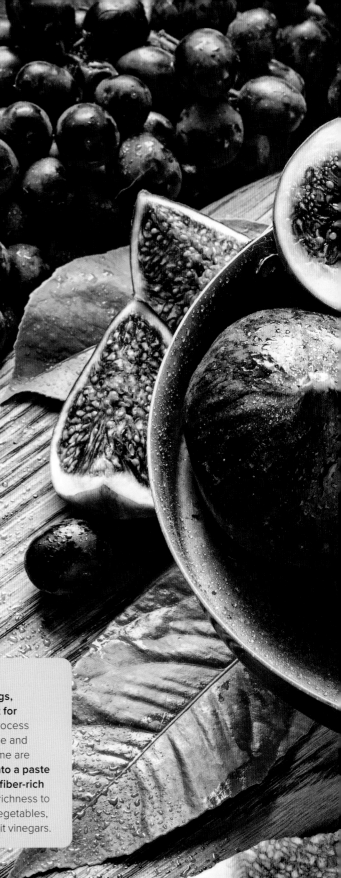

96 | FEEL-GOOD SUPERFOODS

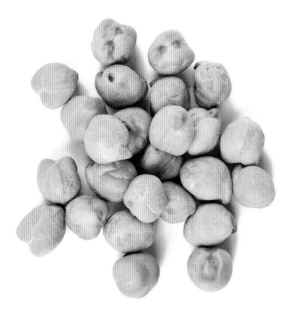

Garbanzo Bean

Enjoy this protein-packed plant food.

Also called chickpeas, garbanzo beans are a staple in the Mediterranean region as well as in India. Their nutlike flavor is delicious, whether you're enjoying whole beans, popular dishes like hummus or crunchy roasted chickpeas, which make a terrific snack. A very nutrient-dense food, just one cup of these cooked beans provides 12.5 grams of fiber, or about half the recommended amount for one day. Like many other beans, they're also a great plant-based source of protein and many nutrients, including manganese, folate and antioxidants.

ALSO TRY If you don't have or don't like garbanzo beans, try other similar beans. Lima beans and northern white beans are mild and creamy and make good substitutes for chickpeas in recipes. Both are similarly excellent sources of fiber and protein.

How to Buy & Enjoy

● **Surprisingly, the process of canning beans actually makes them more nutritious. You can always start with dried beans, but you can also feel good about buying canned (and bagged/boxed) versions of these legumes.** ● When cooking beans in a liquid, be sure to consume the liquid, too—or you'll lose many of the nutrients. You can also let the cooked beans sit in the liquid for up to an hour before serving to reabsorb some of the leached nutrients. ● **Add acidic, sweet and calcium-rich ingredients to beans when cooking them for a long time, to preserve their structure and texture. Molasses and tomatoes combine all these elements, and the flavors pair well with all kinds of beans.** ● Look for various forms of chickpea, including the large, cream-colored version and the smaller, darker version, plus garbanzo flour.

SCIENCE SAYS

Garlic's cancer-fighting potential is especially promising. Research suggests it may reduce the risk of cancers of the digestive tract, including stomach and colon cancer. That's because garlic contains sulfur compounds that may stimulate the immune system's natural defenses.

For optimum freshness, use garlic within 10 days of buying it.

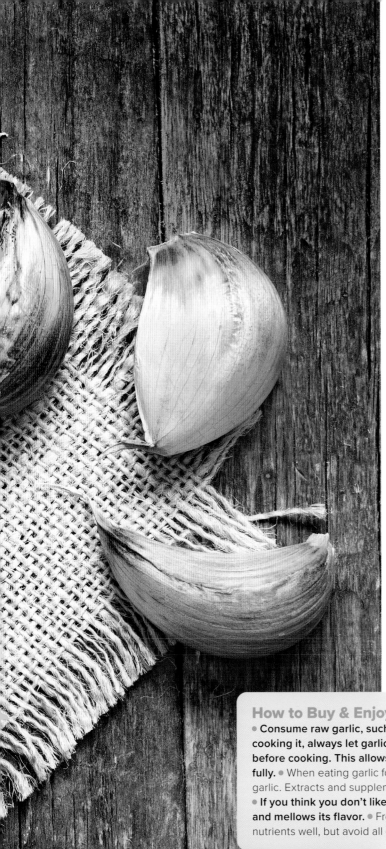

Garlic

A little garlic offers up lots of flavor and preventive nutrition.

The conventional wisdom is right about this herb: Garlic is good for you! And in so many ways, it's amazing. Studies suggest that garlic is good for your heart, may help lower your cholesterol and even fights some types of cancer. Garlic contains many vitamins and nutrients, including vitamin C, B vitamins, manganese, phosphorus and calcium. It's also packed with antioxidants and has antimicrobial properties that can help fight off infection.

ALSO TRY Other members of the allium family, which includes chives, leeks, onions and shallots, have qualities similar to garlic. All have sulfur compounds that give them their pungency, plus the same healthful properties—including potential anti-cancer action.

How to Buy & Enjoy

● Consume raw garlic, such as in pesto, whenever you can. When cooking it, always let garlic rest for 10 minutes after mincing and before cooking. This allows beneficial compounds to develop fully. ● When eating garlic for health benefits, be sure to actually eat garlic. Extracts and supplements aren't as nutritionally effective. ● If you think you don't like garlic, try roasting it, which deepens and mellows its flavor. ● Freeze-dried garlic retains flavor and nutrients well, but avoid all other prepackaged versions.

Grass-Fed Meat

Animals who eat their natural diet of grass, not grain, have healthier fat profiles.

When buying meat from ruminant animals—including beef, bison, goat and sheep—think grass-fed. Traditionally, all those animals have eaten a diet of mainly grass, but in large-scale, industrial agriculture, these animals now eat much more grain. This unnatural diet dramatically alters the nutritional content of the meat. Grass-fed (similar to what's called pastured) products have many more omega-3s, which actually improve heart health—the opposite of the fats you get from grain-fed animals. When buying meat, read label information carefully to be sure the animals were raised on pasture throughout their entire lives. Meat from animals raised on pasture but "finished" on grain will not have the same nutritional content.

ALSO TRY The same principles apply to **pork** and **poultry**. The diet of those animals is more varied than that of ruminants, but they also benefit from pasture. Chickens, for example, get exercise, sunlight and the opportunity to eat plants, insects and other foraged foods. All of this is reflected in the nutrition of the meat and eggs.

How to Buy & Enjoy

● Grass-fed meats cost more to produce than their inferior, commercial counterparts. One way to save money but still include these healthier meat options in your diet is to choose the lower-cost cuts. ● You can also purchase a large quantity of meat directly from a farmer, such as a quarter or half of an animal, in what are called animal shares. You'll probably need a deep freezer to make this option work for you. ● Look for 100 percent "grass-finished" products to get the most nutritional benefits. ● When choosing raw meat, look for signs of freshness with no off smells, but be aware that aged meats can be quite dark—and this doesn't mean they've gone bad. Buy from a butcher counter so you can sniff and ask questions.

The fat in grass-fed meat can actually lower cholesterol levels.

SCIENCE SAYS

While there are many types of grass-fed meat, most available nutrition info centers on beef. Research on grass-fed beef has shown that compared to grain-fed, it has higher levels of omega-3 fats, antioxidants, vitamin A and vitamin E, plus lower levels of cholesterol.

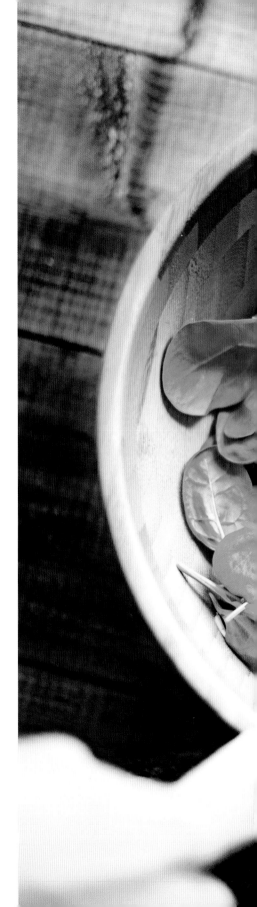

Loose-leaf lettuce

Bok Choy

Greens

All green, leafy vegetables carry boatloads of nutrients.

It's helpful to think of greens as a category—and one to seek out and eat more of, because they are all packed with nutrients. As long as you're eating green, leafy vegetables, you're consuming a low-calorie, nutrient-dense food with tons of vitamins. There are many types to choose from, so mix it up from day to day and week to week. Try lettuce, spinach, cabbage, arugula, kale, chard, collards, mustard greens, tatsoi or bok choy—for starters!

ALSO TRY Turnips, **beets** and **radishes** are typically grown for their roots, but their greens are yummy too. The leafy tops of these root vegetables have similar taste, texture and nutrition to plants like kale, collards and chard. These taste best when picked young and tender.

Arugula

How to Buy & Enjoy

● **To get the most nutritious greens, choose loose-leaf varieties with deep, dark colors.** ● Eat soft and delicate greens raw, and as fresh as possible. ● **Thicker and tougher greens, such as arugula, chard and spinach, can be sautéed or added to stir-fries and soups at the end of cooking.**
● You might enjoy the oldest and toughest greens, such as hardy purple kales, as a cooked dish. Or you can marinate these leaves in salt and an acid, such as lemon juice or vinegar, for 15 minutes before serving them as a salad.

If it's a leafy green vegetable, you'd better believe it's good for you!

SCIENCE SAYS
Studies suggest leafy greens may help protect our brains against dementia. Researchers for the Rush Memory and Aging Project tracked diets of more than 900 older adults. Those eating a serving a day of leafy greens performed better on memory and cognition tests.

Brown and golden flaxseeds are super nutritious.

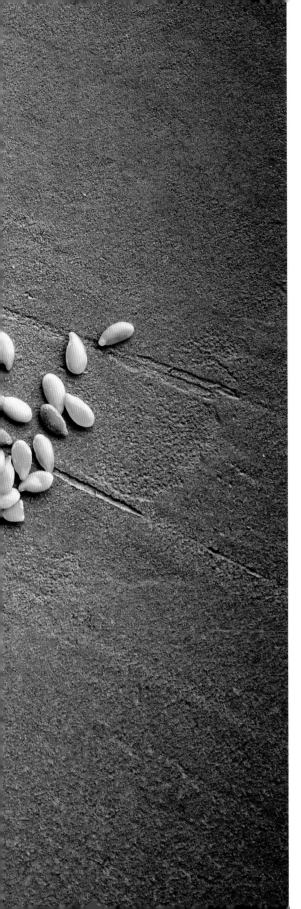

Hemp Seed & Flaxseed

These seeds are packed with nutrients, including protein and heart-healthy omega-3s.

Seeds are almost-plants, full of the nutrients needed to grow big and strong. Their flavors are amped up by roasting and toasting. You can also soak them in water to germinate, unlocking even more goodness. Hemp seeds and flaxseeds are particularly high in protein, fiber, phytochemicals and omega-3s. Hemp seeds are easy: Sprinkle them on any dish that could use a little crunch, or add them to smoothies. Use flaxseeds ground to get the most benefits—it's easy to do in a coffee grinder if you buy them whole.

ALSO TRY Try a variety of **seeds**, like **chia**, **coriander**, **cumin**, **fennel**, **poppy**, **pumpkin**, **sesame** and **sunflower**. Use seed oils for cooking, such as **avocado**, **grapeseed**, **sesame** and **sunflower oils**.

How to Buy & Enjoy

• Although related to marijuana, hemp food products are not from the same plant and can be sold in the U.S. Hemp seeds and oils are widely available. • Store hemp seeds in the refrigerator or freezer to keep them fresh. • **Hemp seeds are easy to use. Sprinkle them on everything, from sweet to savory, to add mild-flavored crunch.** • Flaxseeds are best used in ground form, but the seeds stay fresher if stored whole in the fridge or freezer. You can grind them yourself in a coffee grinder or blender.

Horseradish

This spicy herb is like a leafy, green veggie in disguise.

Horseradish, a member of the mustard family, is a spicy root typically used as a creamy condiment to add flavor to roasted meats and sandwiches. You can buy the mayonnaise-style sauce commercially (usually with additives), but the fresh root couldn't be easier to use. Tuck it in the freezer and grate it over foods to add enormous flavor with minimal calories. Like kale, arugula and broccoli, horseradish is a crucifer and has anti-inflammatory and antimicrobial health benefits.

ALSO TRY Garlic and **wasabi** are also pungent ingredients with cancer-fighting properties. Like horseradish, they add major flavor to food, with few calories.

Skip the jar! Fresh horseradish is a revelation.

How to Buy & Enjoy

● Fresh horseradish is incredible, and a little goes a long way. Buy a root, cut off any greens and keep in the freezer. Grate as needed with a cheese grater or rasp. There's no need to peel the healthy fibrous layer. ● Buy whole, plump roots that aren't dried out. ● Mix grated horseradish with vinegar, for a tangy sauce; with mayo or cream, for a luxe sauce; or with ketchup and lemon juice, to make cocktail sauce. ● Roasting the root, which mellows the complex flavor, is another fine way to use it. ● Think to yourself: What else can I grate this into? Add horseradish to soups, stews, sauces, mashed potatoes or guacamole—basically anything that could benefit from some zing!

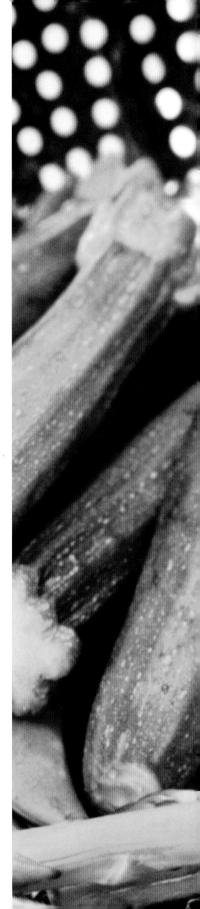

In-Season Veggies

Don't miss out on the ephemeral treats of the garden in the right seasons.

Yes, you can buy almost any green vegetable in stores year-round, but that's a travesty—especially with foods that don't keep well in fresh form. Most foods are better if you buy them in-season, locally. Spring-picked asparagus is tender and delicious, and is one of the healthiest foods on Earth, plus it delivers protein and prebiotics. Fiber-full and nutrient-packed green beans have the best flavor and texture when picked young and eaten quickly. You can even find many amazingly flavored fresh beans in early summer that you may have only ever eaten as a dried bean. Sweet, tiny cucumbers are worth seeking throughout summer if you only know their big, pickled cousins. The skins are nice and thin, which is great, since that's the most nutritious part.

ALSO TRY Some veggies get a nutrient boost when preserved, but most are nutritional duds out of season. **Frozen fruits** are a different story. They'll never be quite as special, but they do retain nutrients well.

How to Buy & Enjoy
- Buy the freshest produce you can find, refrigerate immediately and use ASAP. Shop farmers markets when you can! • **Look for dark green and purple varieties of beans and asparagus.** • Serve raw with dips or shaved into simple salads. Or steam them to preserve nutrients.
- **Toss chopped beans and asparagus into pasta or risotto at the end of cooking.** • Keep an eye out for other seasonal foods, like wild greens in spring, salmon in summer and nuts in the fall.

SCIENCE SAYS

Recent research links gut microflora to cancer, mental health, obesity and more. We introduce helpful bacteria by eating probiotic foods like miso and yogurt. And by eating prebiotics—indigestible compounds in some vegetables like asparagus and tomatoes—we feed the good bugs.

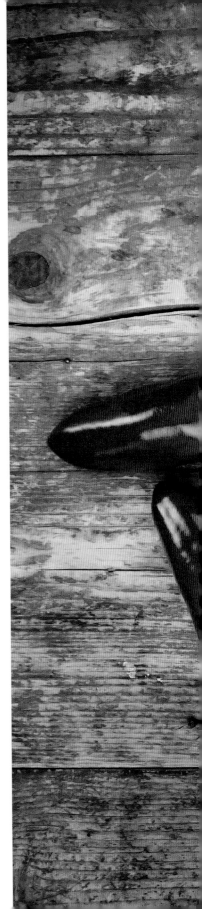

Jalapeño

Hot peppers pack a one-two punch for health and flavor.

Jalapeño peppers are native to the Americas and have long been used (fresh and fermented) to add a spicy kick to many dishes. They're the same species as many other familiar peppers, including bell and cayenne. Jalapeños have a mild flavor and a moderate level of heat compared to some hot chilies. They're also full of antioxidants and a good source of vitamins A, C and K; B vitamins; and manganese. Capsaicin, which is responsible for the heat in peppers, also has anti-inflammatory and antimicrobial power.

ALSO TRY There are many hot peppers to choose from, and all are capsaicin-rich! A few easy-to-find options are **poblano**, **cayenne**, **habanero** and **Scotch bonnet peppers** (see pages 114-115).

How to Buy & Enjoy

- First off, always wear gloves when handling hot peppers! Then wash hands and, even then, be careful not to touch your eyes until you are sure you're in the clear. • You might also like chipotle peppers, which are fully ripened and pickled jalapeños. • Remove hot-pepper seeds to tame the heat—or leave them in for extra spice.
- Jalapeños can be enjoyed raw, but roasting, frying and grilling them improves the sweet-hot-and-acidic flavor.

Fully mature
jalapeños
are red and
ultra-flavorful.

SCIENCE SAYS
Could eating hot peppers
help you lose weight? While
the effect is likely to be small,
some research suggests that
capsaicin could burn a few extra
calories by boosting metabolism.
Perhaps more useful, eating
hot peppers may also act as
an appetite suppressant.

MORE SPICY PEPPERS

Some like it hot—and so should you if you want to add flavor and boost your health.

The fiery seasonings beloved across cultures from India to Mexico enhance flavor in countless curries, hot pots, salsas and beyond. Capsaicin, the compound that makes them hot, works its magic on many levels—from lowering triglycerides to reducing nasal congestion, relieving pain, cleansing out toxins and ramping up metabolism.

HABAÑERO
These little orange pods pack premium heat. About 140 times hotter than a mild jalapeño, they're often found in hurts-so-good chili.

POBLANO
A good grilling pepper that's ideal for stuffing, these hot delights grow fairly big and are usually sold fresh or dried.

SERRANO
Spicier than jalapeño, this fleshy Mexican native has a bright and biting flavor that gives it zest but won't torch your mouth.

CAYENNE
This bright-red pepper is usually consumed dried and powdered as a spice. It's an easy way to add zest—and fat-burning capsaicin.

THAI (BIRD'S EYE)
These little fireballs are popular in Southeast Asian dishes. They're often sold dried, which dials down the heat slightly.

SCOTCH BONNET
This fruity-tasting staple of Caribbean cuisine may sound gentle, but its heat index is quite another story.

ANAHEIM
This large, mild chili is a good starting point for spicy-food newbies. Often used in salsa verde, Anaheims can train the palate for higher levels of hotness.

Kale

This famously healthy food is all that—and much more.

This green lives up to the hype. Nutrient- and antioxidant-rich, kale is also a good source of lutein and zeaxanthin, two nutrients critical to eye health. It's also packed with essential vitamins and minerals, notably manganese; vitamins A, C and K; and B vitamins. One of the best plant sources of calcium, kale is a friend to vegans and anyone with lactose intolerance. Just as important, this leaf tastes great and is versatile. The crunch and texture of raw baby kale leaves is welcome in a salad, but you can also cook any kind of kale. Sauté kale for a side dish; flash-fry or bake into crunchy snacks; simmer in soups; and even pickle it.

ALSO TRY Try other members of the nutritious crucifer crew. Greens: **arugula, bok choy, collard greens, watercress**. Roots: **horseradish, turnip, radish, rutabaga, wasabi**. Others: **broccoli, Brussels sprouts, cabbage, cauliflower**.

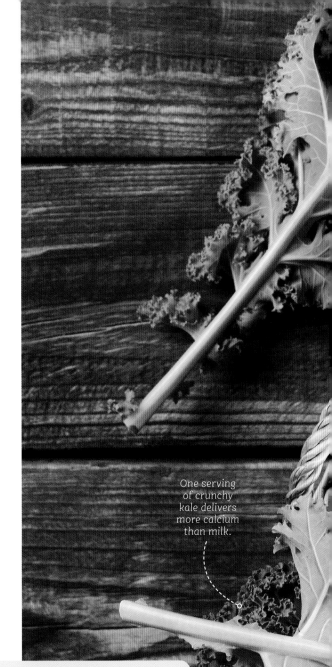

One serving of crunchy kale delivers more calcium than milk.

How to Buy & Enjoy

- Choose fresh bunches with deep color that do not appear to be dried out. The stems should be plump and juicy. These are generally removed when preparing kale, but you can actually roast them and eat them too. Try any of the varieties of kale, and especially the dark-purple ones, which are full of phytonutrients. ● Consider sowing some kale seeds in your yard in the fall, so you can harvest a fresh green salad even in winter. Kale is cold-hardy and incredibly unfussy, quick-growing and easy to manage.
- For salads, use baby kale leaves or look for unfrilly Lacinato or "dinosaur" kale. You can also marinate kale and squeeze or massage it with oil, salt and acid (vinegar or citrus juice) to help soften it. ● For sautéing, flash-frying, baking and adding to soups and stews, you can use any kale variety, no matter the texture.

Lemon

Perk up foods and beverages with a twist of lemon, hold the sugar. But be sure to eat the zest.

We've all heard that vitamin C is good for us—and lemon, like other citrus fruits, is a good source of this essential nutrient. Vitamin C supports the immune system, helps the body absorb iron, and is itself an antioxidant. Where lemon shines is that you don't need a lot of it, and it's a great low-cal way to add flavor to anything and everything. Squeeze a wedge of lemon into water or unsweetened tea instead of having a sweet drink. Try a twist of lemon with meat or veggie dishes for depth of flavor without fat or salt. Lemons are also full of phytonutrients and preserve other foods. In lab studies comparing anticancer properties of different fruits, lemon came in second of all fruits (cranberry was first).

ALSO TRY All citrus is rich in vitamin C. Mix it up with **limes**, **oranges** and **grapefruit.** Have whole fruits, rather than juice, whenever possible—and enjoy that healthy zest.

How to Buy & Enjoy

- **Choose deeply colored, plump fruits with no green spots. Meyer lemons have a sweet flavor and thin peels.**
- The most nutritious part of citrus fruits is the peel. Grate the zest into everything from salad dressings and grilled chicken to pie crust and ice cream. If you aren't going to use it right away, store grated zest in the freezer. Try to buy organic citrus fruits only.
- **Make low-sugar marmalade with a variety of citrus peels. Besides toast, marmalade also adds flavor to meat and seafood. Use pectin designed for low-sugar recipes, such as Pomona's Universal Pectin.** ● Ferment whole lemons with salt to make preserved lemons, a pickled African and Middle Eastern condiment that adds huge flavor to many meals.

119

Lentil

This powerful legume can help you lose weight and may reduce diabetes risk.

Lentils have been uncovered at archeological sites throughout the Mideast. Today, they are consumed all over the world, so there are lots of great recipes. In India, lentils are a staple in vegetarian diets, often prepared as a simple stew. In France, you'll find tiny, tender lentils in salads. There's a lot to like about lentils, which are quick to cook and, unlike beans, don't have to be soaked. Lentils are rich in polyphenols and are an excellent source of protein and fiber. They're also a good source of B vitamins, including folate, as well as iron and magnesium.

ALSO TRY Legumes rich in protein and fiber include **split peas, chickpeas, black beans, kidney beans, cranberry beans, white beans** and **navy beans.**

How to Buy & Enjoy
- Look for lentils that are bright—if they are dull, they are not as fresh. ● They are less digestively problematic than other beans.
- With more than 50 different varieties, you're sure to find a favorite color, flavor and size. Teeny green Puy and French lentils are adored by chefs, because they stay firm when cooked. Red lentils soften considerably, but taste sweeter than others.
- Lentils cook quickly compared to beans, some in just 20 minutes.

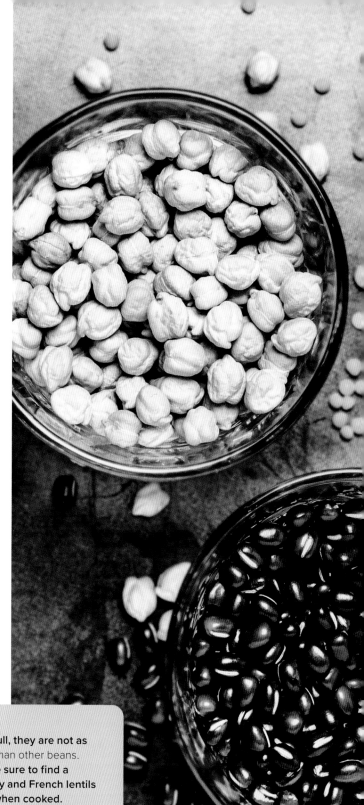

Legumes are a low-glycemic-index food and are often recommended for diabetics. A 2017 Spanish study looked at whether legumes might prevent diabetes. Indeed, researchers found eating legumes of all kinds was associated with a lower risk of developing the disease.

Macadamia Nut

Enjoyed in moderation, this rich nut is part of a heart-healthy diet.

There's a lot to love about this food. Creamy and slightly sweet, macadamia nuts almost qualify as a dessert. They contain respectable amounts of protein and fiber, and are an excellent source of thiamin. Most of their fat is unsaturated. While you could make the case that other nuts have lower levels of saturated fat or higher levels of protein, macadamia nuts still end up a good choice. The FDA recently approved a qualified health claim about macadamia nuts and heart health that can be used on food packaging—no small thing for a food many consider a guilty pleasure.

ALSO TRY **Dark chocolate** and **coconut** are surprisingly healthful properties. If you're willing to splurge on calories and fat, you can do a lot worse than satisfying your cravings for rich food with some of these minimally processed, plant-based treats.

How to Buy & Enjoy

● Freshly harvested macadamia nuts are a true joy. If you find yourself on a tropical island, be sure to get some! ● The flavor of macadamia nuts goes a long way. Chop them up to sprinkle over soups, salads and vegetables. ● Finely chopped macadamias also make an amazing crust for chicken and fish fillets. ● To make nut butter, blend salted or unsalted macadamias in a food processor using the pulse button, adding coconut oil, as needed, for texture.

Maitake

Mushroom

Delicious gourmet mushrooms are among the most medically useful foods you could ever eat.

Wood ear

Matsutake

Shiitake

Many popular culinary mushrooms also have health benefits. Shiitake, maitake, matsutake and wood ear mushrooms appear to be especially potent, in addition to being deeply flavorful. Mushrooms readily lend their strong flavors to fats and liquids, so one way to save money is to use small quantities in recipes like risotto and beef stew. All mushrooms are good sources of fiber, antioxidants, magnesium and potassium and boast much more protein, vitamin D and B vitamins—nutrients mainly obtained from animal foods—than other produce. (To maximize vitamin D, mushroom growers have to be sure to expose them to sunshine or a particular kind of ultraviolet light.) Mushrooms also have many applications in herbal medicine, where they really shine at boosting the immune system. Many species also are being studied for their ability to inhibit tumor growth.

ALSO TRY Few foods are as widely used in herbal medicine as mushrooms; two that stand out are **garlic** and **turmeric**, both featured elsewhere in this guide.

SCIENCE SAYS

Research suggests mushrooms can stimulate the immune system. In a 2014 study, maitake and shiitake extracts stimulated the immune systems in mice, both individually and when extracts from the two mushrooms were administered together.

Save the tough stems to make nutritious mushroom stock.

How to Buy & Enjoy

● Frozen and dried mushrooms cost less than fresh. Drying them intensifies enzymatic activity and flavor, and they are easily reconstituted in hot water. Strain and use the soaking liquid to cook rice, pasta and soups. ● Mushroom is one of few foods that improves somewhat in flavor after harvest, up to about four days—but unless you're gathering them yourself (and know what you're doing), what you get in stores probably has reached that point, so use them quickly.

● Store mushrooms loosely in a partially closed container, with a towel tucked in to absorb moisture. Contrary to popular opinion, it's fine to wash them—but do so just before use. ● Some mushrooms, such as morels and plain white button mushrooms, contain a mild toxin that disappears with heat. Be sure to cook them.

WHITE BUTTON
This common variety has a particular carbohydrate that stokes the metabolism and maintains blood sugar levels. They're also high in disease-fighting selenium.

CREMINI
These young portobello mushrooms, often known as "baby bellas," offer similar weight-loss benefits and are also good sources of vitamins B6 and B12.

MORE EXOTIC MUSHROOMS

Go beyond buttons and give your taste buds a treat with these disease-fighting varieties.

With almost no calories, the goal is more, more, more when it comes to enjoying mushrooms! To help get your daily fix, whisk baby bellas into eggs in the a.m., toss up a maitake-and-wild-rice salad for lunch or sauté some shiitakes for a satisfying dinner, with—or in place of—meat.

PORCINI
Meaty and similar to the portobello, the porcini contains potent anti-inflammatory properties that may decrease the symptoms of asthma.

PORTOBELLO
Their dense texture and umami flavor makes them a great meat substitute or sandwich-bun replacement.

CORDYCEPS

Supplements and products with cordyceps extract have become popular for their ability to deliver energy to the muscles, especially during exercise.

SHIITAKE

These umbrella-shaped brown caps have greater quantities of cancer-preventing properties than other mushrooms.

MAITAKE

Also known as Hen of the Woods, maitakes contain beta-glucans, which have several anti-cancer functions. They can also reduce some of the side effects of cancer treatments.

DID YOU KNOW?

People who replaced meat with mushrooms for four meals each week lost 13 pounds in five weeks.

REISHI

These orange, red and brown fungi contain gandodermic acid, which helps reduce cholesterol and lower high blood pressure.

OYSTERS

Whitish, fan-shaped oyster mushrooms may have therapeutic effects against breast and colon cancers. They're also high in antioxidant compounds.

There's no
end to the flavor
combos you
can use with
meaty mussels.

Mussel

Among shellfish, mussels stand out as an affordable option and a good source of omega-3s.

Mussels are a great addition to your cooking repertoire. They're a good source of omega-3 fats, especially relative to other shellfish. They are also a good source of protein, B vitamins, zinc and iron. And perhaps best of all is that they are more affordable than almost all other shellfish, widely available and incredibly simple to prepare. They're also well-suited to an aquaculture environment, so farming mussels presents fewer environmental challenges than raising many other types of fish.

ALSO TRY Like mussels, **oysters** are high in omega-3 fats and both oysters and **clams** are bivalves, which many suggest makes them a good choice for aquaculture, because their production has a benign impact on the environment.

How to Buy & Enjoy
• Purchase fresh mussels with their shells closed. • When you get home, scrub the shells under cold water with a clean brush.
• Look for tiny hairs poking through the shells and pull hard to remove these "beards."
• If, after cooking, any mussels remain closed, discard them.

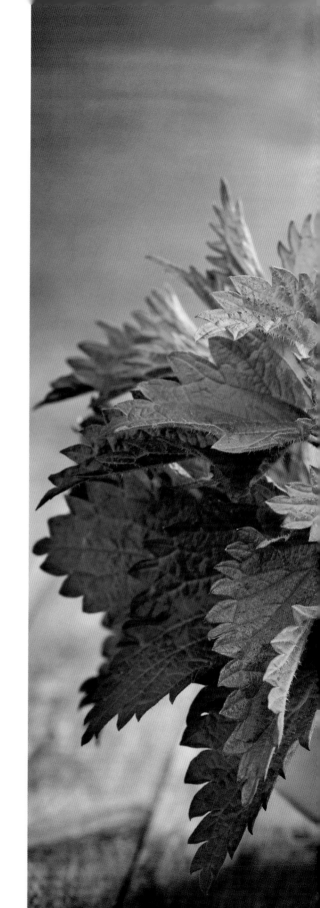

Nettle

This plant, frequently considered a weed, is actually a highly nutritious green vegetable.

Finding and cooking stinging nettles require a little bit of work, but many people find them well worth the effort. This wild plant is full of nutrients, including vitamin A, calcium and iron, as well as antioxidants. It has a long history of use as both a food and an herbal medicine. For fresh nettles, if you can't find them for sale, your best bet may be planting them in a garden. (Many people harvest these and other edible plants from the wild, but that's not safe unless you know what you're doing.) It's also smart to read up on nettle's medicinal and culinary uses before cooking with this potent plant. For example, some experts recommend against consuming nettles during pregnancy.

ALSO TRY **Dandelion greens**, **purslane** and **lamb's quarters** are also frequently considered weeds, but they can be wild-harvested or grown intentionally for their excellent nutritional properties.

How to Buy & Enjoy
● **Look for bright-green nettles with short, tender stems.** ● Always wear gloves when working with stinging nettles—during harvest and kitchen prep. ● **Never eat nettles raw; treat them as a cooking green instead. You can cook and eat the flowers, too.** ● For most preparations, you can treat nettles just like spinach. Sauté them in olive oil; or blanch them in boiling water for a few minutes, then drain and chop them up to add to other dishes.

SCIENCE SAYS

A 2013 article in the International Journal of Food Science found cooked stinging nettles to be a good source of essential nutrients. A 100-gram serving meets 90 to 100 percent of your daily need for vitamin A, and also provides calcium, iron and protein.

Use nettles as you would any cooking green, or try them in a tea.

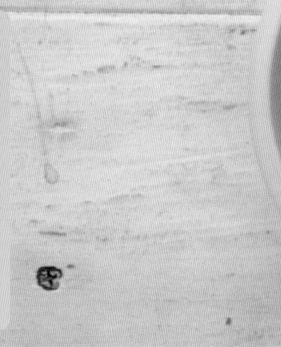

Olive Oil

Polyphenol-rich olive oil also has healthful fats and is the most useful cooking oil.

A high-quality olive oil is delicious when used simply as a dip for bread or to make salad dressings. Mild and buttery in flavor, olive oils are perfect for cooking almost anything. You can even use them in cake recipes. Olive oil is a supremely healthy choice for its high levels of polyphenol antioxidants. Essential to the famously healthy Mediterranean diet, olive oil has been the subject of a wealth of research associating it with a reduced risk of heart disease and diabetes.

ALSO TRY When you need a neutral flavor, you can also use **sunflower oil**, another minimally processed, plant-based cooking fat.

How to Buy & Enjoy

- Look for extra-virgin olive oil from the first pressing, ideally with a specific location and date of harvest included on the label. You can use this unadulterated cooking fat for all purposes, even frying. For neutral needs, such as in a cake recipe, use olive oil from later pressings labeled as "light" or "mild." ● For maximum flavor, try some of the special varietal olive oils made from a single variety, such as Castelveltrano, Coratina, Kalamata, Koroneiki and Mission. ● Olive oil that is green in color is produced when unripe olives are used at harvest. Green olive oil generally contains a higher level of polyphenol and has a more robust taste than gold or yellow olive oil.
- Light and heat destroy beneficial compounds and produce off flavors in olive oil. Buy in dark containers; store in a dark spot away from heat. The fresher, the better: Use a bottle within the first year after harvest.

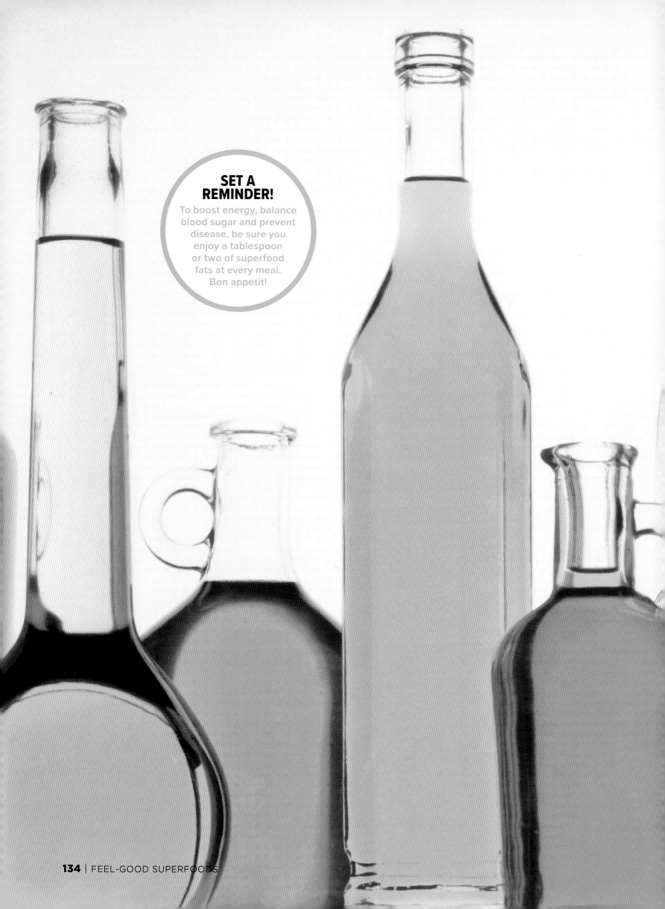

SET A REMINDER!

To boost energy, balance blood sugar and prevent disease, be sure you enjoy a tablespoon or two of superfood fats at every meal. Bon appétit!

THE WORLD'S HEALTHIEST OILS

In general, always choose cold-pressed, unrefined
extra-virgin oils that were harvested recently (within the previous year
is best). Better brands will have this information on the label.

OIL	IN THE KITCHEN	TO COOK OR NOT
AVOCADO	Mild flavor; safe at high temperatures; be sure you're buying unrefined	Either
COCONUT	Rich; satiating; slight coconut taste; solid at room temperature (and thus spreadable)	Either
FLAXSEED	Mildly nutty flavor; keep in refrigerator	No
HEMP SEED	Dark green oil with a strong, distinctive taste; OK in salad dressings, but better drizzled on cooked vegetables; keep in refrigerator	No
NUT	Fine flavors and aromas of almond, hazelnut, macadamia and walnut oils are beloved by chefs; excellent in salad dressings	No
OLIVE	Wide range of memorable flavors (mild, fruity, grassy, peppery, etc.); always choose extra-virgin, recently harvested and low in acidity—check labels; save prized olive oils for finishing dishes (the stronger the flavor, the higher in nutrients)	Either
PUMPKIN SEED	Great for heart, skin, prostate, immune system, cholesterol profile; best variety is from 'Styrian Hulless' pumpkins	No
SACHA INCHI	Rich peanutty flavor; best source of omega-3s	No
SESAME SEED	Toasted version has strong, distinctive and addictive flavor; can be used with other oils to enhance overall flavor without overpowering	Either
SUNFLOWER	Neutral flavor; withstands high temperatures; relatively inexpensive; good all-purpose cooking oil	Yes

Add nutritious
onion skins
to simmering
water for
an easy broth.

Onion

This kitchen staple is valued for its anticancer, antioxidant and prebiotic properties.

Onion is a familiar kitchen ingredient, used to add flavor to all kinds of dishes—but it's amazing how many healthful properties it has. Onions contain vitamin C, especially raw, as well as fiber, B vitamins, manganese and antioxidants. Onions also have prebiotic compounds, which they retain even after they are cooked, so eating onions can help support beneficial bacteria in the digestive tract. There are many traditional medicinal uses for onions, but in modern research they are especially valued for the anticancer action of their sulfur-containing compounds.

ALSO TRY It's not just onions. All alliums have sulfur-containing compounds that are associated with anticancer action. Try **chives**, **garlic**, **leeks** and **shallots**.

How to Buy & Enjoy
● All onions are nutritious; you'll get the most benefit from eating them raw. To tame spicy onions, marinate them in water with a splash of lemon juice or vinegar, then rinse.
● Onions that smell and taste strongest are healthiest, with red and yellow types being far more nutritious than "sweet" onions. ● All onions sweeten with heat. You might as well choose yellow and red onions for cooking in order to get the biggest antioxidant bang. ● Choose onions with intact peels so you can eat the nutrient-dense layers closest to the outside of the bulb.

SCIENCE SAYS

A 2015 review of anti-cancer research on onions and other allium family members concluded that eating them may decrease cancer risk. The strongest protection may be for the GI tract. The anti-cancer benefits are likely from their bioactive sulfur compounds.

A 2017 study in the U.K. found that free-range and organic eggs had more vitamin D3 than eggs from hens raised indoors, likely because of greater access to sunshine. Organic regulations in the U.S. and U.K. aren't identical, but both require birds have access to the outdoors.

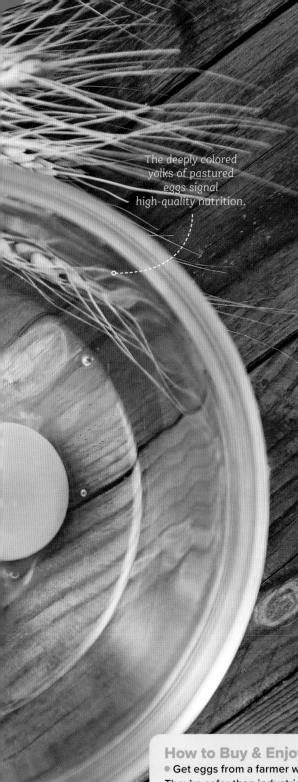

The deeply colored yolks of pastured eggs signal high-quality nutrition.

Organic Egg

Choose eggs you know are from hens eating a healthy diet with access to the outdoors.

For many of us, eggs are a regular part of our diets and they're essential to numerous dishes from flan to frittata. Eating eggs was once thought to increase cholesterol, but recent research suggests dietary cholesterol doesn't impact cholesterol levels as much as other factors, such as the type of carbohydrates we eat. So cholesterol in eggs is no longer a big concern. Eggs are a good source of protein, selenium, phosphorus and A and B vitamins. They're also one of the few natural food sources of vitamin D. When you choose organic eggs from pastured hens, you also know that the hens were raised on grass and supplemented with organic feed but no antibiotics, pesticides, hormones or synthetic fertilizers.

ALSO TRY **Sustainably raised, pastured eggs** from local farms. When you buy certified organic eggs, you can find the standards they were certified to meet, but that comes with a hefty price tag. A dozen organic eggs can cost nearly double the price of commercial eggs. However, many small producers meet and often exceed these standards but choose not to seek official certification. To buy eggs from small producers, try your closest farmers market.

How to Buy & Enjoy
● **Get eggs from a farmer who doesn't scrub off naturally protective membranes. They're safer than industrial eggs (important for raw-egg recipes).** ● Eggshells (like butter) are semipermeable. Use this to your advantage by tucking aromatic herbs or a little truffle oil into the container. ● **Avoid sulfur flavors in eggs by using low heat, no matter what kind of eggs you're making—and don't oversalt them.**

Plum

Fresh plums are a juicy treat, while dried plums are both useful in the kitchen and good for the digestive system.

All types of fresh plums are good sources of vitamin C and other antioxidants. The Australian Kakadu plum actually is the best source of vitamin C on Earth, with 50 times that of an orange. Plums also have vitamins A and K, and smaller amounts of several other nutrients. When dried into prunes, they lose most of the vitamin C, but other nutrients, such as fiber, vitamin K and potassium, become more concentrated. Prunes have many health benefits, including improved digestive function and stronger bones. Despite the benefits, watch how many you eat: Not only do prunes have a lot of natural sugar, they're also a natural laxative.

ALSO TRY   Other stone fruits, such as fresh **peaches**, **apricots** and **nectarines**, are all good sources of vitamins A and C and fiber—and all of them become super high in fiber when they are dried.

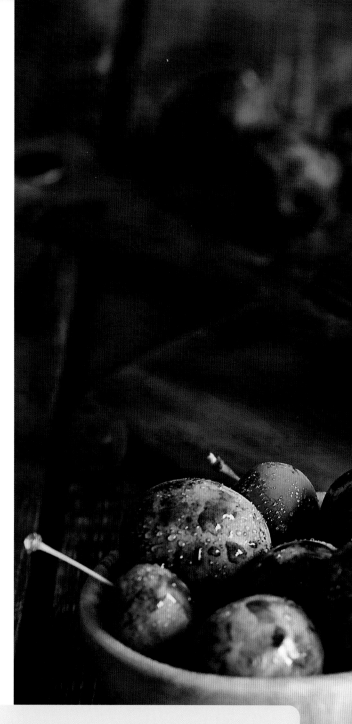

How to Buy & Enjoy

● You may be surprised at the range of plums at farmers markets and orchards. Look for the candy-like Autumn Sweet, which is great for fresh eating, or intensely tart Damsons, perfect for stewing. ● Choose plums with blue, black and dark-red skins for the most antioxidants—and eat those skins! ● Shop for plums in late summer and early fall to enjoy the sweetest types. ● Leave plums on the counter to ripen. Once ripe, refrigerate them, and eat within five days. ● Dried plums have a surprising number of uses. Include them in braises, where they slowly break down, adding a sweet-tart complexity to the liquid. No one will know you put prunes in your baked chicken or beef stew!

SCIENCE SAYS

Multiple studies looking at bone strength in postmenopausal women have found that regularly consuming dried plums is associated with strong bones and less loss of bone density. In a 2016 study, positive effects were linked with eating as few as six prunes per day.

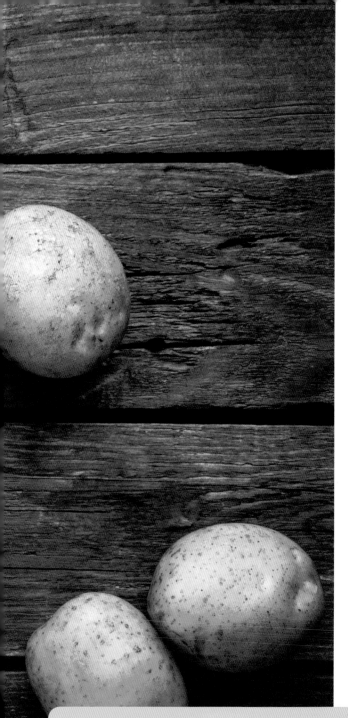

Potato

This standby is packed with potassium—and don't skip the skin!

Potatoes are an important staple around the world. They're a good source of carbohydrates that can help you feel full and also contain vitamin C, iron, B vitamins and more potassium than bananas. To get the most nutrition out of a potato, put down the peeler. The skin is where many of the nutrients are concentrated, and it's an added source of fiber. Fried potatoes are definitely *not* a great option, especially if fried in low-quality, trans fat–loaded oils that are continually reheated (such as how they're prepared at fast food restaurants). But eaten with a little bit of healthy fat, as part of a nutritious meal, potatoes are a great whole food. Choose blue and purple potatoes for an added bonus of anthocyanin antioxidants.

ALSO TRY Like white potatoes, **sweet potatoes** contain potassium, vitamin C and B vitamins. In addition, they have even more vitamin A than regular potatoes.

How to Buy & Enjoy

● For maximum beneficial compounds, choose small and colorful potatoes whenever possible. To boost nutrition further, reduce the impact to your blood sugar by eating potatoes with some type of fat and vinegar, or refrigerating them after cooking to eat the next day. ● Many people have never eaten a freshly dug potato, but it's incredibly flavorful and tender. It's worth checking farmers markets in spring and fall— and definitely worth growing some of your own. ● New potatoes (also called waxy potatoes) have less of an impact on blood sugar compared to baking potatoes. They also make great potato salads. ● Store potatoes in a cool, dark, ventilated location.

BURDOCK ROOT
This natural detoxifier is great for the liver and can help with skin problems like acne and eczema.

MORE TUBERS AND ROOT VEGETABLES

These starchy and sweet veggies are deeply satisfying choices for diabetics and anyone who wants to lose weight.

Root vegetables and tubers are among the most nutritious foods on earth, packed with antioxidants, vitamins and minerals. They are considered to be slow-burning carbs, delivering consistent energy while helping you feel full. Plus, many root vegetables can satisfy a sweet tooth! Try some of these superfood options.

BEETS
The antioxidant pigments in beets, known as betalains, show great promise for the prevention of cancer.

YACÓN
Sweet yacón contains a sugar called inulin that boosts digestion and healthy gut bacteria while keeping blood sugar stable.

CARROTS
Besides keeping eyes healthy, the provitamin A in carrots boosts immunity, heart health and cancer prevention.

MACA ROOT
Powerful Peruvian maca root is shockingly nourishing. It supports adrenal and hormone function, endurance and stamina.

RADISHES
The spicy flavor in radishes comes from compounds that prevent the formation of cancer cells.

JERUSALEM ARTICHOKES
Jerusalem artichokes, or sunchokes, are "prebiotic": They stimulate growth of useful bacteria in the digestive system.

CELERY AND PARSLEY ROOTS
Celery and parsley plants both have edible roots and are delicious served raw in salads.

Pumpkin Seed

This tasty seed is a good source of magnesium, zinc and iron.

Packed with nutrients, toasted pumpkin seeds are a pretty perfect whole-food snack. They are good sources of magnesium and zinc, as well as iron and vitamin E. Eat them without the shells if you prefer; consumed this way, they're called pepitas. But you can also eat the shells for extra fiber and crunch. For added flexibility, you can even chop up or grind pumpkin seeds to use them as toppings or as an ingredient in baked goods.

ALSO TRY Sunflower seeds are another good choice for snacking or for sneaking a few added nutrients into meals when you sprinkle them on as a topping. Like pumpkin seeds, sunflower seeds are good sources of magnesium, zinc and vitamin E.

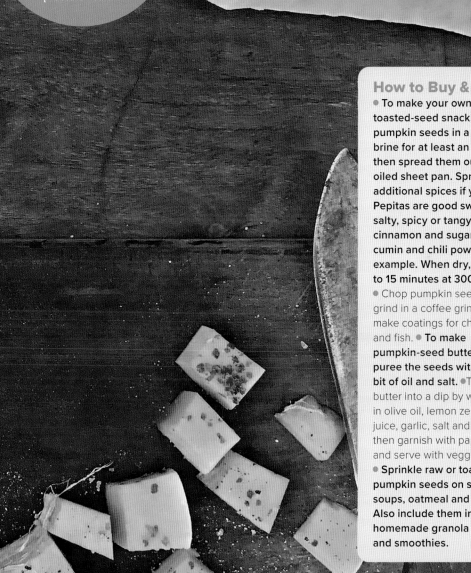

How to Buy & Enjoy

● To make your own toasted-seed snack, soak pumpkin seeds in a salty brine for at least an hour, then spread them out on an oiled sheet pan. Sprinkle on additional spices if you like. Pepitas are good sweet, salty, spicy or tangy. Try cinnamon and sugar, or cumin and chili powder, for example. When dry, bake 10 to 15 minutes at 300°F.
● Chop pumpkin seeds or grind in a coffee grinder to make coatings for chicken and fish. ● To make pumpkin-seed butter, simply puree the seeds with a little bit of oil and salt. ●Turn the butter into a dip by whirring in olive oil, lemon zest and juice, garlic, salt and pepper, then garnish with paprika and serve with veggies.
● Sprinkle raw or toasted pumpkin seeds on salads, soups, oatmeal and yogurt. Also include them in homemade granola and smoothies.

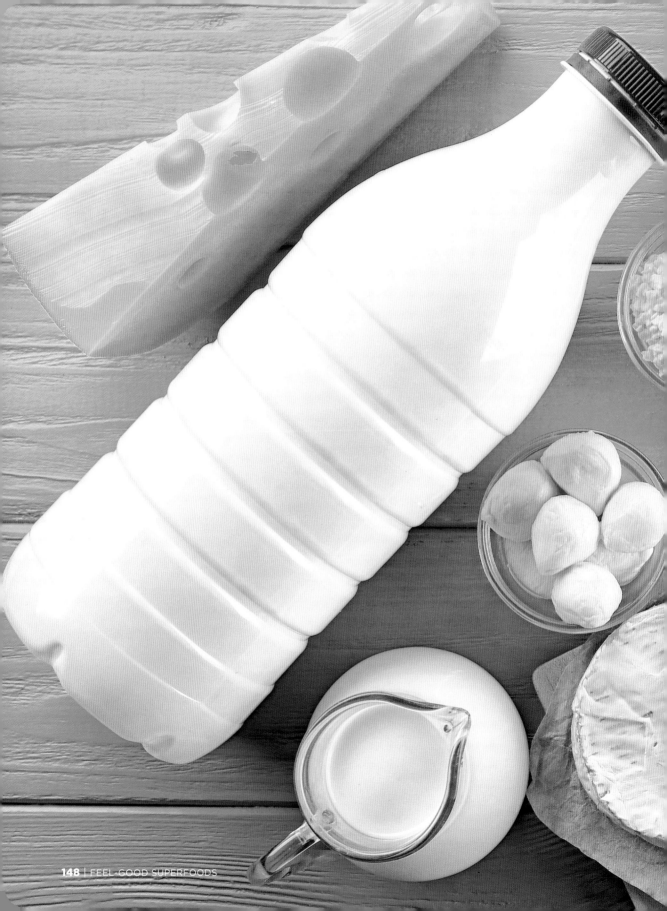

Quality Dairy

Choose organic or pastured dairy to get more of those healthy fats.

Most people know milk is great for its calcium, but it's also rich in protein and B vitamins. And if you can find dairy products from animals raised on pasture, their products have higher levels of healthy fats, especially an important one called CLA. Look for products certified as pastured through organizations such as the American Grass-Fed Association. Another option is to buy organic dairy, which requires natural forage for dairy animals during at least part of the year. That tells you the animals were raised at least partially outside, rather than in full-confinement operations, and that the milk is not from animals given antibiotics or other hormones.

ALSO TRY Vegetarian? Some of the best plant sources of calcium are vegetables in the cabbage family, including **kale** and **broccoli**. For omega-3s, flax and **hemp seeds** are both excellent plant sources.

SCIENCE SAYS
A 2016 analysis of 170 studies found organic milk to have significantly higher levels of polyunsaturated fats and omega-3s than conventional milk. Many of the studies were European, and organic standards there require that animals get more food from pasture.

How to Buy & Enjoy
● Many people like raw milk for nutritional benefits that come from eating foods in their natural state. Raw milk can be delicious and nutritious, but you have to be certain your source is impeccable. You can also pasteurize it yourself by simmering at 145°F for 30 minutes. Also look for raw-milk cheeses, because during the cheese making process, potentially unsafe microbes are outcompeted by the fermentation cultures. ● The next closest thing to raw milk is pasteurized (not "ultrapasteurized" or "ultra-heat-treated") but not homogenized milk. Homogenization benefits the dairy industry, not the consumer. If you're not bothered by seeing a layer of luscious cream at the top of the jug, you'll get better-tasting milk with better texture. To make skim milk, skim the cream off the top and reserve for other uses. ● Explore the world of quality dairy, including yogurt, kefir, skyr, cream cheese, crème fraîche and, of course, cheese.

Quinoa

This grain has something for everyone, including those on vegetarian and gluten-free diets.

This flavorful, healthy food comes from South America, where thousands of varieties are grown. Quinoa is a seed, but for nutritional purposes, it's easiest to think of it as a grain. It can be used in place of rice or pasta, but it also makes a good breakfast cereal. Quinoa contains all the amino acids to make it a complete protein, useful for people seeking plant-based protein. It's also gluten-free and nutritionally dense. Quinoa is a good source of not only protein but also fiber, manganese, magnesium, phosphorus, B vitamins and iron.

ALSO TRY Whole grains of all kinds contribute to a healthy diet. The main thing to look for is unprocessed grain—the aim is to get as many nutrients from the original grain as possible. In processed grains, many of those nutrients have been stripped away. In addition to quinoa, look for other grains that are easy to cook and consume in their whole form, such as **bulgur**, **amaranth** and **teff**. (See pages 152-153.)

This tasty seed may help you lower your cholesterol.

SCIENCE SAYS

A 2015 review of research on quinoa found many benefits. For example, this exceptionally nutritious plant may act as a prebiotic, encouraging beneficial gut bacteria. Quinoa can also be grown in a range of conditions, which could make it useful in places with food scarcity.

MORE ANCIENT GRAINS

See ya, pasta: Add more nutrition and flavor to your next meal with these whole grains.

Ancient grains are actually just whole grains that haven't been modified or cross-bred by modern agriculture. That makes many of them naturally gluten-free and a hearty, flavorful alternative to traditional wheat.

MILLET
The nutty-tasting little gems are a delicious gluten-free stand-in for wheat—and a great source of plant protein (6 grams per cup) for vegetarians.

BULGUR
Light, chewy and high in manganese, magnesium and iron, bulgur wheat is also rich in protein and fiber.

KAMUT
Similar to bulgur, kamut has up to 40 percent more protein than common wheat, making it a high-energy substitute.

TEFF
The tiny kernel (about the size of a poppy seed), is gluten-free and loaded with calcium—more than any other grain.

FARRO
Higher in fiber than most other grains, farro is super filling and an excellent source of magnesium and iron.

SPELT
This almond-shaped grain contains some gluten, but less than traditional wheat, and is often used as a substitute for white or wheat flour.

AMARANTH
This mainstay of the Aztecs packs more protein than any other ancient grain and can help lower cholesterol.

SCIENCE SAYS

Raspberries have high levels of polyphenols. These antioxidants have potential benefits in combating serious illnesses such as heart disease, cancer and diabetes. For specific benefits of raspberries, new research is encouraging but, so far, limited to animal and cell studies.

Raspberry

Sure, they're tasty, but did you know that raspberries are crazy high in fiber?

All berries are packed with vitamins, minerals and antioxidants, and raspberries are no exception. They're also good sources of vitamins C and K and manganese. They get their color from antioxidants called anthocyanins. But raspberries really stand out when it comes to fiber. A single cup has almost one-third of your daily need for fiber (and more than you'd get from a bowl of oatmeal). They are a perfect fresh snack, besides being a great topping. The most nutritious varieties grown today are Caroline, Heritage Red, Summit, and all types of black raspberries. Golden raspberries are significantly lower in antioxidants.

ALSO TRY **Strawberries** and **blackberries** are in the same family as raspberries. Blackberries have almost as much fiber, and all berries are good sources of antioxidants. Be on the lookout for **black raspberries**, which have many more times the antioxidant content of red raspberries—and have shown remarkable anticancer abilities in lab studies.

How to Buy & Enjoy

• Raspberries don't stay fresh long, so try to get them locally grown and recently harvested. They're not hard to grow, either, and homegrown raspberry canes can keep producing for a decade or more. Plus, they'll produce many canes you can give to friends to start their own patch. • You can extend the life of raspberries a little bit by swirling them gently in water with a splash of vinegar. Lay on a towel to dry, then store in a single layer in the crisper drawer. • Raspberries also freeze beautifully. Open-freeze them with a very light dusting of sugar in a single layer on a sheet pan. When frozen solid, transfer to storage containers. • When buying raspberries, check that they are aromatic (floral-smelling), deeply colored, plump, soft and juicy-looking but not leaking juice out yet (that means they're overripe).

Rosemary

Add this Mediterranean herb to foods for its flavor, its aroma and an extra helping of antioxidants.

Rosemary is a popular herb native to the Mediterranean. It's a wonderful low-calorie flavor enhancer for meat, vegetables and baked goods, and is also often consumed as a tea. Rosemary contains nutrients such as vitamin C, iron and fiber, though because you don't eat much at one time, these are present in small amounts. However, rosemary is also full of antioxidant compounds. Traditionally, this herb is associated with memory; and, interestingly, some research suggests the scent of rosemary can slightly boost performance on cognitive tests.

ALSO TRY Some of the most popular culinary herbs are closely related to rosemary, and likewise, are full of nutrition and antioxidants. **Basil**, **thyme**, **sage** and **oregano** are also members of the mint family. One characteristic of this family is that it has highly aromatic plants, so these herbs can all add appetizing scents as well as flavor to your meals!

A little rosemary goes a long way, but you can use it in a surprising number of recipes.

How to Buy & Enjoy

● **Rosemary is one of the few herbs that remains potent when dried, and there's nothing you have to do but leave it open in the fridge—it'll dry nicely. It also grows in crummy soil with little moisture, and there are a few varieties that will survive cold winters even if you don't bring the pots inside. These are just a few of the reasons to grow your own rosemary for year-round use!** ● Hold on to the stems. After you've stripped the leaves off, you can turn the sturdiest stems into skewers for kebabs or throw them on a fire simply to enjoy the wonderful aroma. ● **Rosemary is the first herb to flower in spring, and you can garnish dishes with the pretty blue buds.** ● Rosemary is a famous partner to roasted meats, but it's also good with seafood and in baked goods. Rosemary goes particularly well with fall fruits, nuts and chocolate.

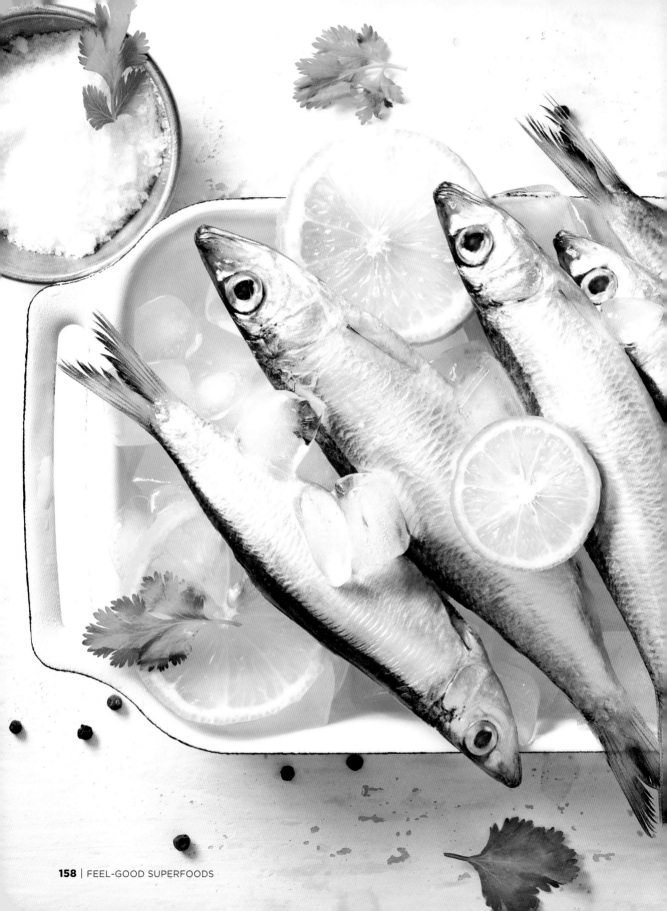

Sardine

This tasty little fish is a good source of both omega-3 fatty acids and vitamin D.

Sardines are a good addition to your diet, whether you buy them canned or are lucky enough to find them fresh. They're a smart source of omega-3s, specifically DHA and EPA, which most of us could use more of. Regularly eating these healthy fats is linked to reduced risk of conditions like heart disease and dementia. Sardines are also good for protein, vitamin D, B vitamins and calcium.

ALSO TRY Other small fish, like **anchovies** and **mackerel**, are low on the food chain and therefore sustainable, plus they're low in mercury and high in omega-3s.

How to Buy & Enjoy

● Sardines and other herring-family members are high in healthy fats that can generate "off" flavors, which is why they're often canned, smoked and salted. ● However, fresh sardines are amazing. They should smell of the sea, not "fishy," and should be used quickly. Sardines flash-frozen after being caught and thawed close to use also are great. ● Try to find a quality fish merchant. Look for whole fish. Precut fish should be glossy, without browning or sliminess. Rinse before use and pat dry. ● To prepare whole sardines, coat in olive oil, salt and pepper and broil for 5 minutes.

Sauerkraut & Kimchi

Pickled cabbage is full of vitamin C and probiotics. Just watch the overall sodium content.

Homemade sauerkraut is one of the simplest possible dishes—it's made with just salt and cabbage, and allowed to ferment naturally. Kimchi is a more complex take on the same idea: Napa cabbage is fermented but with added flavorings like garlic, ginger and red pepper. In either case, when the pickling is done through the souring and preserving process of fermentation (not with vinegar, which also acts as a preservative), you're getting a live-culture food, which means it adds probiotics (good bacteria) to your diet. Both sauerkraut and kimchi can also be good sources of vitamin C and B vitamins.

ALSO TRY Look for other foods labeled as containing live cultures. These can include **yogurt**, **kefir**, **skyr**, **miso**, **kombucha**, **hot sauce**, **soy sauce**, **tempeh** and many types of **pickles**.

How to Buy & Enjoy

● When shopping for fermented foods, be sure to buy brands that contain live cultures. Many brands will instead have been pasteurized, which kills probiotic bacteria. ● Use a little bit of the brine from sauerkraut and kimchi in cooking liquids—or blend with sunflower oil, Dijon mustard and a smidge of honey to make an easy salad dressing. ● Serve sauerkraut and kimchi as condiments, especially alongside tender, fatty foods. Their crunch and tang also complements burgers and sandwiches. ● Use leftover brown rice to make a nutritious fried-rice breakfast incorporating kimchi, eggs, leftover veggies and greens.

Tea

From ancient China to modern salons, there's no matching the legacy and benefits of a cuppa.

Tea has been famously used to tell fortunes, inspire poetry and even incite war. But its role in traditional medicine may be the most enduring. For centuries, people have believed that tea has curative powers, including the ability to purify the body and preserve the mind. It has been used for detoxification and as a natural remedy for everything from cancer to heart disease. Remarkably, in recent decades, thousands of published studies have offered scientific proof that many long-held health claims about tea are medically sound.

SCIENCE SAYS

While green tea often steals the spotlight, numerous studies show that all types of tea can play a significant role in lowering the risk of a vast number of conditions, including heart disease, stroke, cancer and obesity. Its benefits are generally attributed to flavonoids and related polyphenols, as well as the antioxidant catechins.

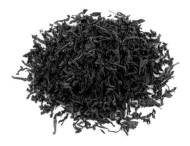

BLACK TEA

Study after study shows that drinking black tea improves cardiovascular health—and the more you drink, the more your heart benefits! Researchers at UCLA found that people who regularly consumed three or more cups of black tea per day had a 21 percent reduced risk of stroke compared to those who skipped it.

GREEN TEA

It can fight cancer, lower cholesterol and boost immune function. But the most exciting benefit may be this brew's ability to melt pounds. Compared to other teas, green tea has slightly higher levels of catechins, specifically EGCG, which rev up metabolism and shrink fat cells, particularly in the abs. In one study, people who drank green tea burned an extra 70 to 100 calories a day. Another showed that people who drank green tea and caffeine lost an average of 2.9 pounds during a 12-week period while sticking to their regular diet.

OOLONG TEA

Scientists say oolong is easier on the stomach than green tea and actually contains more polyphenols. They also say that just one cup of oolong increases metabolism by 20 percent for two hours—nearly twice as long as three strong cups of green tea.

ROOIBOS TEA (RED TEA)

Technically not a tea but a tisane, rooibos is made from the leaves of the red bush plant from South Africa. It's caffeine-free and notable for its ability to literally stop flab from forming. According to South African researchers, the polyphenols and flavonoids in this red brew inhibit the formation of new fat cells by as much as 22 percent. Plus, it can benefit exercise performance, improve concentration and boost mood.

WHITE TEA

Because of the gentle way it's treated and the minimal processing involved, this delicate, light-colored tea retains much higher levels of antioxidants than green tea, meaning it can do much of what green tea can, only better! A German study published in the journal *Nutrition & Metabolism* showed that white-tea extract caused fat cells to break down, while preventing new fat cells from forming.

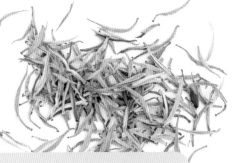

How to Buy & Enjoy

● **Tea has the same benefits whether you drink it hot or iced, so feel free to enjoy it year round.** ● There are four varieties of true teas—black, green, white and oolong—all originating from the same plant. Oxidation, processing and other factors give each brew its own distinctive color, flavor and unique health benefits. ● **Herbal teas are not considered true teas—instead, they are called tisanes.**

Tomato

Who doesn't love a fresh tomato? But this summer star may be even better for you when cooked.

Tomatoes are such an important staple in so many parts of the world that it would be hard to avoid them completely, even if you wanted to. Fortunately, they're good for you. Tomatoes are good sources of vitamins A, C and K and contain fiber, potassium and manganese. They're full of antioxidants, especially lycopene, a carotenoid found in red fruits. Interestingly, cooking tomatoes appears to increase their total antioxidant activity.

ALSO TRY While tomatoes are especially rich in the antioxidant lycopene, they're not the only source. It's also found in other red-pigmented fruits, including **guavas**, **watermelon** and **grapefruit**. The more red you see in the flesh, the more lycopene it has.

How to Buy & Enjoy
- Fresh, in-season tomatoes are better for you when prepared with fat. Drizzle with your best olive oil and a pinch of salt. The salt amps up the sweet and acid flavors in tomatoes; the oil helps your body absorb all those nutrients.
- Cooking tomatoes, either via sauce-making, ketchup-making or canning, is another way to supercharge the tomato nutrition. ● When tomatoes are not fresh and abundant at the market, you can still enjoy them. But instead of buying hard, unripe, flavorless tomatoes in December, you'll be better off enjoying sun-dried and canned tomatoes to get true summer flavor. ● Try the many varieties of heirloom tomatoes, which are gorgeous but also range in flavor from pineapple and lime to chocolate and pepper. The options are endless!

How to Buy & Enjoy

● Use turmeric as a culinary spice. Turmeric is also available as a supplement—but before taking it, talk to your health-care provider. ● Keep turmeric root in the freezer and grate it with a box grater or rasp as needed. There's no need to peel away the nutrient-rich skin when grating finely. (Use ginger and horseradish in the same way.) ● **Turmeric adds color, citrus aroma and a slightly sharp flavor to dishes. Use in curries, mustard and pickle recipes and to add color to rice and grains.** ● To make soothing golden milk, simmer turmeric with ginger, peppercorns and winter spices in milk or nut milk with a little honey for about 10 minutes. Strain and serve warm.

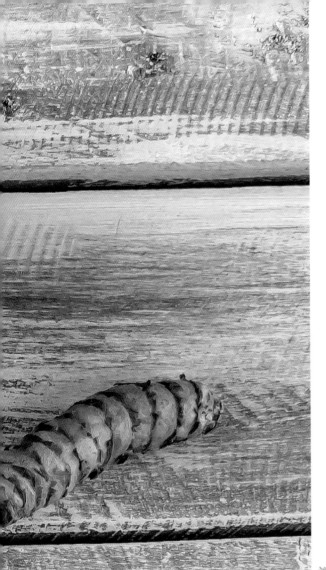

Turmeric

This health-promoting rhizome adds spice and antioxidants to your meals.

Turmeric is one of the main ingredients in curry powders, and this increasingly popular spice has other culinary uses. You can even enjoy it as a beverage, such as golden milk or turmeric tea. Turmeric is anti-inflammatory and contains curcumin, a potent antioxidant. Some people also find that turmeric helps soothe the stomach. Also, like most spices, it's an excellent low-cal way to add flavor to foods without adding salt, fat or sugar in the process.

ALSO TRY Like turmeric, **ginger** is a rhizome, a popular culinary spice and a good source of antioxidants. Enjoy these spices alone or in dishes together, as they often appear.

This vibrant powder offers more than just crazy color.

SCIENCE SAYS
Turmeric has abundant medicinal potential being actively studied, with many researchers investigating how to make the powerful compound curcumin more bioavailable in medicines. Meanwhile, you can enjoy this exotic spice in a number of culinary ways.

SCIENCE SAYS

A 2016 study in Nutrition Research and Practice found that mice fed a high-fat diet supplemented with brown seaweed had reduced markers of inflammation. Those fed kombu, in particular, had lower insulin resistance than those fed the high-fat diet without seaweed.

Mineral-rich toasted seaweed provides all the comforts of snacking, with its natural saltiness.

Undersea Superfood

Seaweed comes in a variety of tastes and textures, all full of vitamins and especially minerals.

Seaweed is also called sea vegetable and macroalgae. Not all types of seaweed can be eaten, but there are many delicious varieties, including wakame, kombu, nori and dulse. Red seaweeds like nori are particularly high in protein. Seaweed also contains fiber, antioxidants and numerous vitamins and minerals, including iron, calcium, magnesium and manganese. Seaweed is rich in iodine, which is beneficial in small amounts but needs to be handled carefully by anyone who suffers from thyroid problems.

ALSO TRY While there's really nothing quite like seaweed, if you can't get it (or just don't like it), **kale** may be the next best thing. This leafy, green vegetable is not only full of vitamins and minerals, but the many different types of kale—from common to Lacinato and Chinese—provide a variety of textures, from chewy to crispy, that make it versatile in the kitchen. Also, homemade baked or fried kale chips taste remarkably like the seasoned seaweed snacks you can buy in the store.

How to Buy & Enjoy

- **Make your own seaweed snacks by rubbing dried nori with oil and salt, then toasting it quickly in a hot, dry cast-iron pan.** • To improve digestibility of gas-producing foods, add kombu to simmering pots of beans and soup. Discard before serving. • **Sprinkle any of the many tasty dried seaweeds over salads to boost flavor and nutrition.** • Use large sheets of roasted seaweed to wrap up sandwich and salad fillings for a quick, nutritious lunch.

Vinegar

Use this basic ingredient to bring out
the best in healthful whole foods.

Vinegar has at least 5 percent acetic acid, which gives it many useful culinary properties. Vinegar is not typically used in large enough quantities to be a good source of particular vitamins and minerals. Instead, think of vinegar as a seasoning tool that can help you cut out overly salted and sugared processed foods. Vinegar truly is a fundamental pantry ingredient you'll use all the time, if you learn to cook from scratch. Use it to brighten flavors and make quick pickles, salad dressings and sauces.

ALSO TRY **Lemons** and **limes** are key ingredients to keep in your pantry. They add acidity and bring out the flavor of all your healthiest dishes—such as salsa, guacamole, fish and roasted vegetables.

How to Buy & Enjoy
- **Often, when something doesn't taste quite right, people reach for salt or maybe sugar or more butter. Many times, the element of taste missing is actually acid. Try adding vinegar to brighten dishes. It also helps cut cloying sweetness, powerful bitterness and unpleasant greasiness.**
- You'd be wise to spend money on a few quality vinegars rather than stocking numerous types. You are well-stocked if you have decent vinegars made from cider, rice, wine and sherry. ● **Infuse your own vinegars with garden-fresh flavors by steeping veggies in narrow-necked bottles of vinegar.**
- Make quick-and-easy pickles: Simply cover veggie slices in vinegar and refrigerate.

SCIENCE SAYS

A 2013 article based on the famous Nurses' Health Study found walnut consumption to be associated with lower rates of type 2 diabetes in women. When analyzing dietary patterns over time, women who ate the most walnuts also had the lowest rates of diabetes.

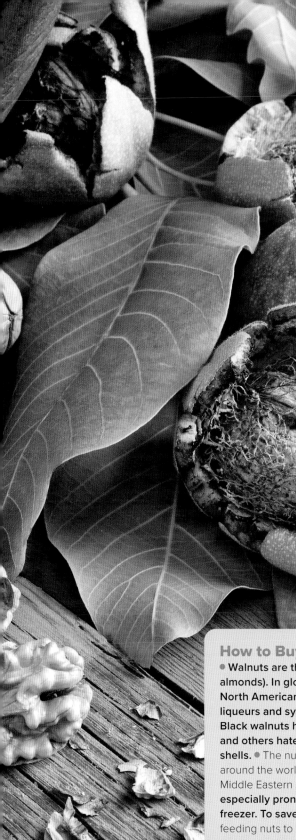

Walnut

English walnuts and many other tree nuts are full of polyunsaturated fat.

Nuts in general are nutrient-dense foods. While high in calories, walnuts and many other nuts are also packed with nutrients and have healthy fat profiles. English walnuts are a good source of fiber, protein, B vitamins, copper and manganese as well as antioxidants. Walnuts are a heart-healthy choice; they contain mostly polyunsaturated fat, which includes a lot of those beneficial omega-3s. Walnut oil carries these benefits too, compared to other vegetable oils.

ALSO TRY Many other tree nuts have high levels of unsaturated fats and may help promote heart health as part of a healthy diet. Consider **almonds, hazelnuts** and **pecans** (turn page for more).

How to Buy & Enjoy

● Walnuts are the second-most widely consumed nut in the world (after almonds). In global cuisine, they're used in many ways that differ from North American uses, such as in walnut milk and sticky-sweet walnut liqueurs and syrups. English walnuts are most common and are sweetest. Black walnuts have a distinct, astringent flavor that some people love and others hate, and they are more difficult to extract from their sticky shells. ● The nutty-bitter flavor of walnuts makes them foundational in sauces around the world, including garlicky Italian pasta sauce and sweet and tangy Middle Eastern sauces featuring pomegranates and peppers. ● **Walnuts are especially prone to rancidity. Buy fresh when possible and store in the freezer. To save money, buy pieces instead of halves.** ● Use caution when feeding nuts to children who may not yet know whether they have allergies.

MORE NUTS AND SEEDS

Tiny but mighty, these superfoods are basically real-food multivitamins.

Nuts and seeds are the embryos of new plants, which means they possess the indispensable ingredients necessary to make life. They are full of vitamins and trace minerals and contain the fats that help your body absorb these nutrients—plus protein for energy and fiber to keep you full. Nuts are a self-contained super-snack and seeds are easy to add to almost any dish, sweet or savory.

PINE NUTS
Pine nuts have the highest protein content of any nut.

PEANUTS
A quarter of every peanut (technically a legume) is pure plant protein.

PECANS
Pecans increase metabolism.

FLAXSEEDS
Consuming ground flaxseeds feeds the beneficial flora in your gut.

MACADAMIA NUTS
Macadamia nuts help metabolize fat.

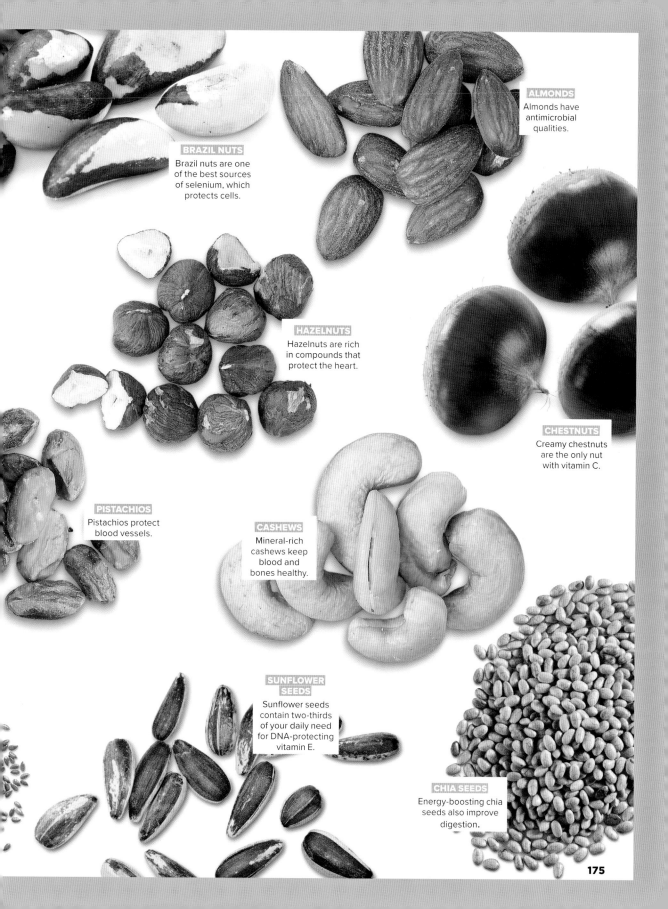

BRAZIL NUTS
Brazil nuts are one of the best sources of selenium, which protects cells.

ALMONDS
Almonds have antimicrobial qualities.

HAZELNUTS
Hazelnuts are rich in compounds that protect the heart.

CHESTNUTS
Creamy chestnuts are the only nut with vitamin C.

PISTACHIOS
Pistachios protect blood vessels.

CASHEWS
Mineral-rich cashews keep blood and bones healthy.

SUNFLOWER SEEDS
Sunflower seeds contain two-thirds of your daily need for DNA-protecting vitamin E.

CHIA SEEDS
Energy-boosting chia seeds also improve digestion.

Wild Rice

Enjoy the deeper flavor of this
alternative to white rice.

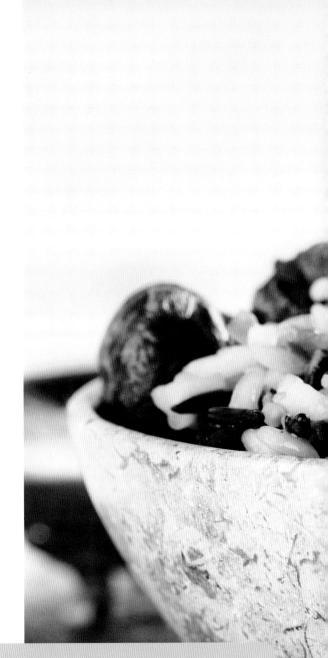

Wild rice is native to North America, where it's
a traditional food of Native American and First
Nations groups who gather it via canoe from the
Great Lakes region. You can still find truly wild,
traditionally harvested rice from this area. However,
most commercially available wild rice is now
cultivated in Minnesota, in California and as far
away as Australia. Wild rice, a reedy aquatic plant
with complex flavor, is a very distant cousin of
the plant we usually call rice. It has more flavor,
and also more protein. It's also full of antioxidants,
fiber, B vitamins and minerals, including zinc,
phosphorus and manganese.

ALSO TRY **Brown rice** is another great
option when you need a grain base. Studies
have suggested that replacing white rice with
brown rice can cut diabetes risk.

How to Buy & Enjoy
● You can buy hand-harvested wild rice directly from Native American businesses in the Great Lakes
region. Look for "hand-harvested" or "lake rice" instead of cultivated wild rice. It comes with a high price
tag, but you can reduce cost by enjoying it blended with other rice and grains; this works nicely, since
wild rice has more flavor and texture. ● Wild rice contains about twice as much moisture as other kinds of
rice. Processing it requires parching it, which lends the already earthy, floral flavor a nutty complexity—much
like aging tea does to fresh, green tea leaves. The process also gives it a chewy texture and makes cooking
time longer. A pressure cooker comes in handy, but you can also presoak wild rice for several hours in
warm water. ● Wild rice is great on its own as a side dish, and it can be used in breads and casseroles or
stuffed into roasted mushrooms, peppers, tomatoes or zucchini. ● Wild rice is a classic ingredient in soups
because it retains some of its chewy character after other ingredients have gone to mush.

SCIENCE SAYS

Fish-consumption guidelines are confusing, but wild-caught salmon comes out looking pretty good. Experts suggest we regularly eat fatty fish high in omega-3s to reduce the risk of heart disease, among other benefits, with salmon often cited as an example that's also low in mercury.

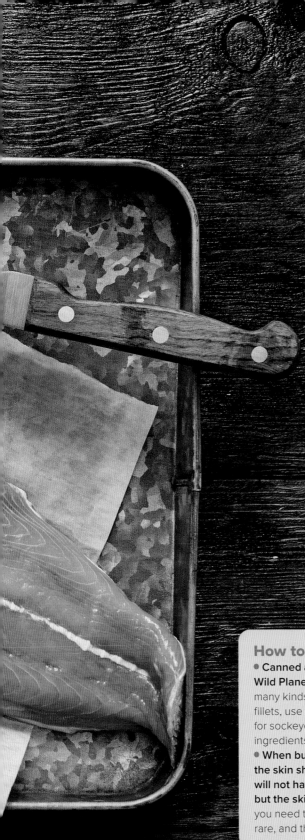

Wild Salmon

This delicious fish is a good source of protein and nutrients.

Most health advice will tell you to enjoy a variety of fish—and wild salmon is one to add to the mix when you can. In addition to omega-3 fats, wild salmon is also a good source of protein, and it's also full of other nutrients, including B vitamins, potassium and selenium. What's the difference between farmed and wild salmon? Environmentalists strongly prefer wild salmon as more sustainable than other aquaculture practices. And chefs tend to prefer wild salmon for its superior flavor.

ALSO TRY Other fish high in omega-3s and low in mercury include **anchovies** and **sardines**. Check out fda.gov/fishadvice for specifics on mercury.

How to Buy & Enjoy

● Canned and foil-packed salmon can be great, and new brands like Wild Planet are canning only sustainably caught wild fish. ● There are many kinds of salmon from many places, typically named by origin. For fillets, use the best fresh or frozen fish you can find. Look especially for sockeye, king and wild Atlantic salmon. For dishes with many ingredients, use less-expensive types or quality packaged salmon. ● When buying fresh or thawed fish, make sure the meat is moist and the skin shiny. It should smell of the sea, not "fishy." Salmon often will not have been scaled, so you may have to scrape them away— but the skin is delicious. ● Wild salmon is leaner than farm-raised, so you need to be careful when cooking it. Anything more than medium-rare, and the fish will become tough and very dry.

Xtra Superfoods

Boost the super-quotient in all of your meals with these healthy toppings, flavorings and mix-ins.

When you're learning about purchasing healthy foods, words you may hear frequently are "avoid added..."—as in, avoid added sugar, salt, fat, preservatives, stabilizers, dyes and artificial flavors. But here are a few extras you can *add* to foods that only increase flavor and nutrition. Add these to smoothies, juices, yogurt, vegetables, soups, salads and baked goods. You can even sprinkle them into popcorn and onto breakfast cereal.

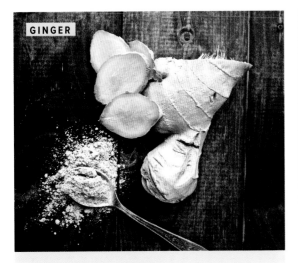

GINGER

How to Buy & Enjoy
- Look for ginger that has thin, shiny skin and a pungent, spicy smell. Avoid any knobs with thick, fibrous skin or soft spots. Store roots in freezer (with peels). Use cheese grater or rasp to grate (peels included) into all kinds of dishes to boost their anti-inflammatory power.

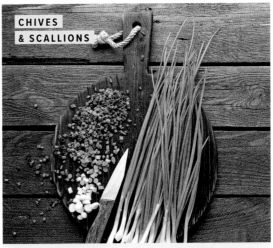

CHIVES & SCALLIONS

How to Buy & Enjoy
- Add immune-boosting alliums like chives and scallions to most any savory dish. Grow chives in a sunny window for a year-round supply. Look for scallions with vibrant green tops and lengthy white stalks. Store scallions in water to keep them growing as you keep snipping.

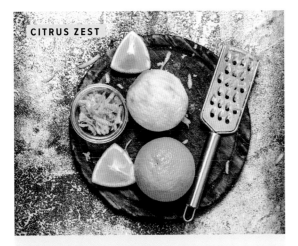

CITRUS ZEST

How to Buy & Enjoy
- Most people throw away citrus rinds, but they're the healthiest part! Use a rasp to grate washed zest off all citrus fruits, then store it in the freezer to sprinkle over sweet and savory foods. You can also mix it with a tiny bit of granulated sugar to create flavored sugars.

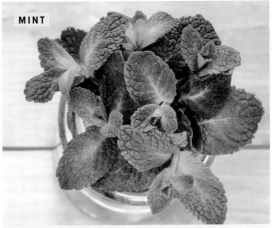

MINT

How to Buy & Enjoy
- Soothing mint has been shown to ease nausea, aid in digestion and help fight fatigue. Keep mint for up to a week by storing in a plastic bag, loosely wrapped with a damp paper towel. Use it to flavor your tea or water, or chop it up and sprinkle over veggies instead of salt.

Yogurt

This tangy, fermented food
is a good source of probiotics,
protein and calcium.

Chosen carefully, yogurt can be a great addition
to your diet. It's a good source of protein and an
excellent source of calcium, among other nutrients,
including zinc and B vitamins. It's also one of the
best food sources of probiotics, those live cultures
that help maintain good digestion. The main thing
to watch out for is sugar; but plain, full-fat yogurt
is a healthy choice. Greek yogurt is just strained
yogurt. It is higher in protein but also lower in
calcium than regular yogurt.

ALSO TRY **Kefir** is another live-culture, tangy,
fermented milk product that can potentially have
benefits for digestive health. It's thinner than most
yogurts and is typically enjoyed as a drink. As
with yogurt, look out for added sugar. **Skyr** is also
a lot like yogurt, but is made from a much tangier
bacterial culture. Skyr is almost always accompanied
by fruit to balance the incredible tartness. Siggi's
is a wonderful, widely available brand.

How to Buy & Enjoy

● **Buy yogurt that says it contains active live cultures. If you don't tolerate dairy,
try many other kinds of yogurt, such as those made from almond, cashew or
coconut milk, that also contain these beneficial live cultures.** ● Most of the
zillions of yogurts available in grocery stores contain additives and tons of sugar.
Seek out plain, full-fat yogurt for the best flavor, texture and nutrition. Add your
own honey, fruit or jam at home, and you'll still end up with a healthier choice.
● **You can also put yogurt to savory uses, such as in cooling sauces to go with
spicy dishes or by substituting yogurt for mayo or cream cheese in recipes.**
● If you have a great milk source near you, definitely try making your own yogurt.
It's shockingly simple—find any number of recipes easily available on line.

SCIENCE SAYS

There's still a lot to learn about probiotics, especially how gut microorganisms affect overall health. It's not yet clear what benefits eating live-culture foods might offer people who are healthy. However, research suggests these foods may help those with digestive problems, especially problems related to antibiotics use.

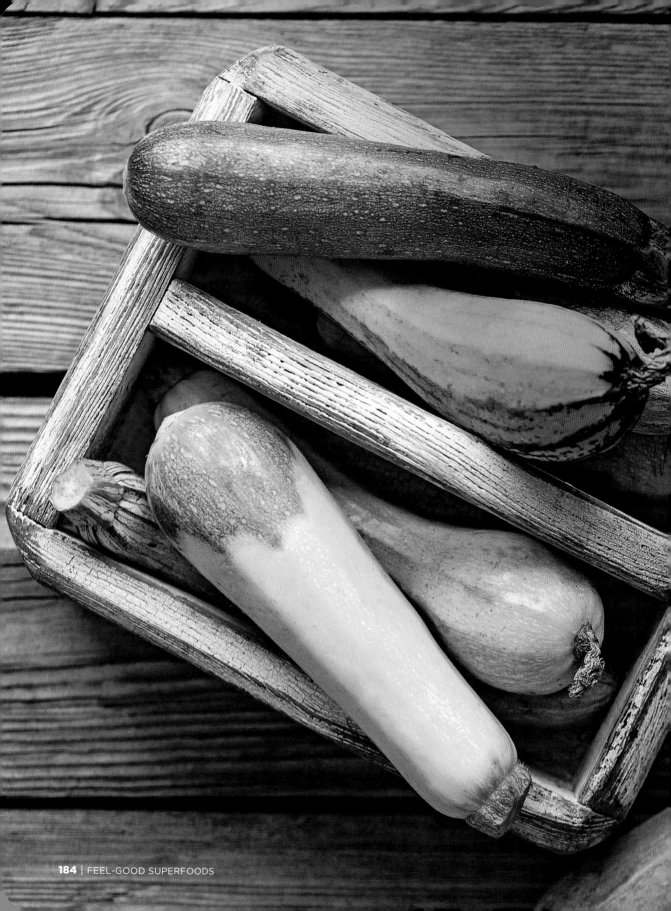

Zucchini

Look for new ways to enjoy this summer standby to get more produce in your diet every day.

Zucchini and summer squash are so abundant in the warm months that they're cheap, with friends and neighbors sometimes literally giving them away. Cooked squash is a good source of vitamin A; it also contains vitamins C and K, fiber, and minerals such as potassium and manganese. Take advantage of this summer bounty and work squash into all kinds of vegetable sides; breads and other baked goods; and raw salads and vegetable trays with dip. You can even use them as zucchini noodles, or "zoodles." Let all the creative ways people have come up with to use an abundance of zucchini inspire you to work more vegetables into your overall diet.

ALSO TRY Be sure to mix up your vegetables and get some from all categories. U.S. dietary guidelines break it down as follows: **dark-green vegetables**, **red and orange vegetables**, **beans and peas**, **starchy vegetables** and all other vegetables. Learn more at choosemyplate.gov/vegetables.

How to Buy & Enjoy

● **Look for the many wonderfully flavored Italian zucchini varieties at farmers markets. Smaller zucchini and squash also are more flavorful—as well as more nutritious.** ● Grated zucchini and squash can add bulk, moisture and nutrients to baked goods, such as classic zucchini bread. To remove extra moisture, simply salt the zucchini and pat it dry. ● **That never-used horizontal slicer on your cheese grater can shave zucchini into thin ribbons that make nice salads. Toss with olive oil, lemon juice and salt and pepper.** ● Slice zucchini lengthwise, stuff with quinoa, top with hard cheese and bake.

INDEX

A

Acai berries, 70–71, 83
Almond butter, 75
Almonds, 173, 175
Amaranth, 150, 153
Anaheim pepper, 115
Anchovies, 159, 179
Ancient grains, 150–153
Antioxidant-rich foods, 22
Anxiety, 61
Apricots, 140
Artichokes, 72–73
 Jerusalem, 145
Arugula, 116
Avocado, 74–75
Avocado oil, 107, 135

B

Bad (saturated) fats, 51
Baked kale chips, 40
Banana, frozen, 42
Barley, 76–77, 150
Basil, 156
Beans, 16, 19, 34, 65, 78–79, 98–99,
 120, 129
Beet greens, 104
Beets, 144
Berries. See also individually
 named berries
preventing mold on, 83
 recommended daily intake, 18
Bison burger, 43
Black beans, 78–79, 120
Black tea, 163
Blackberries, 82, 96, 155
Blackcurrants, 80
Blood pressure, reducing, 60
Blueberries, 60, 80–81, 83
Bok choy, 116
Brain function, 22
Brazil nuts, 175
Breakfast, 33
Broccoli, 67, 116

Brown rice, 60, 150, 176
Brussels sprouts, 116
Buffalo wings, healthier swap for, 43
Bulgur, 150, 152
Burdock root, 144

C

Cabbage, pickled, 160–161
Calcium, sources of, 26
Calories, myths about, 48
Camu Camu berries, 83
Candy bars, healthier swap for, 42
Cantaloupe, 67
Carbohydrates
 healthier food swaps for, 41
 myths about, 52
Carrots, 144
Cashew butter, 75
Cashews, 175
Casu marzu (cheese), 65
Cauliflower, 41, 116
Cayenne pepper, 112, 115
Celery root, 145
Cereals, whole-grain low-sugar, 76
"Certified organic," USDA definition,
 56–57
Cheese, 84–85
Cheetos, healthier swap for, 40
Chestnuts, 175
Chia pudding, 42
Chia seeds, 107, 175
Chicken wings, grilled, 43
Chickpeas, 98–99, 120
Chile peppers, 65, 112–115
Chipotle pepper, 114
Chives, 101, 136, 181
Chocolate pudding, healthier swap
 for, 42
Citrus fruits, 118–119, 181
CLA fat, 149
Coconut, 86–87, 93, 122
Coconut oil, 135
Coffee, 88–89

Collard Greens, 116
Color, phytochemicals and, 14, 16
Complex carbohydrates, 52
Cordyceps mushrooms, 127
Coriander seeds, 107
Cottage cheese, 85
Cranberries, 82
Cranberry beans, 120
Cremini mushrooms, 126
Cumin seeds, 107

D

Daily food intake, recommended,
 14–16
Dairy products, 33, 148–149
Dandelion greens, 130
Dark chocolate, 42, 60, 90–91, 122
Dates, 86, 92–93
Depression, fast foods and, 60
Detoxification, liver, 59
Diabetes, type 2, 60
Diet, improvement strategies,
 30–35
Digestion, 22
Dinner, 33
Distracted eating, 33

E

Eating healthily. See Healthy eating
Eating out, weight gain and, 34
EBCG catechin, 60
Egg yolks, 65
Eggplant, 94–95
Eggs, 34
 distinguishing fresh from old, 65
 organic, 138–139
 80/20 Plan, 58–61
Elderberries, 80
Energy, foods improving, 62
Energy bars, 56

F

Farro, 153

Fats, 33
  bad vs. good, 5
    CLA, 149
    myths about, 50
    Feeling hungry, 33
Fennel seeds, 107
Fermented foods, 33, 160–161
Feta cheese, 85
Fiber, 26, 52, 60
Figs, 86, 93, 96–97
Flavor, adding, 46
Flaxseed, 106–107
Flaxseed oil, 135
Focus, foods improving, 62
Folate, sources of, 26
Food
  healthier swaps/choices, 40–43,
  44, 47. See also Healthy eating
  labeling explained, 54–57
  as medicine, 11, 58
  nutrient-dense, 48
  preserving freshness of, 38, 83
  recommended daily intake, 14–16
Food journal, 32
Food waste, reducing, 38
Freshness, preserving, 38, 83
Frozen foods, 38, 110
Frozen treats, 42, 56
Fruits, 33, 46
  berries, 70–71, 80–83
  citrus, 118–119
  organic, 39
  recommended daily intake, 15, 16
  stone fruits, 140–141

G
G-BOMBS, 17–19
Garbanzo beans, 98–99
Garlic, 100–101, 108, 124, 136
Garnishes, for added nutrition, 46
Ginger, 167, 181
Gluten sensitivity, 61
Goat cheese, 85

Goji berries, 70
Goldenberries, 82
Good (unsaturated) fats, 51
Granola, healthier swap for, 41
Grapefruit, 119, 164
Grapeseed oil, 107
"Grass-fed," defined, 57
Grass-fed meat, 102–103
Green tea, 58, 60, 88, 163
Greens, 104–105, 116, 130–131
  recommended daily intake, 19
Grilled wings, 43
Growing your own food, 38
Gruyère cheese, 84
Guava, 164

H
Habanero pepper, 112, 114
Hamburger, healthier swap for, 43
Hazelnuts, 173, 175
Headaches, 61
Healing powers, 22
"Health food," caveats about, 54–57
Healthy eating
  basics of, 8–29
  food costs and, 36–39
  strategies for, 30–35
Healthy plate model, 16
Heart-friendly diet, 60
Heartburn, 61
Hemp seed, 106–107
Hemp seed oil, 135
Herbs, 33, 38
Hiding healthy ingredients, 46
Hippocrates, 58
"Hormone-free," defined, 57
Horseradish, 108–109, 116
Hot sauce, 160

I
Ice cream, healthier swap for, 42
Immune system/Immunity, 22, 60
In-season vegetables, 110–111

Insomnia, 61
Iron, sources of, 26

J
Jalapeño pepper, 112–113, 114
Jefferson, Thomas, 67
Jerusalem artichokes, 145
Journaling, about your food, 32

K
Kale, 67, 116–117, 169
  baked chips, 40
  liver detoxification and, 59
Kamut, 152
Kefir, 160, 182
Kidney beans, 79, 120
Kimchi, 160–161
Kombucha, 160

L
Labeling, terms used in, 56–57
Lamb's quarters, 130
Leafy greens, 104–105, 116, 130–131
  dark, liver detoxification and, 59
  recommended daily intake, 17
Leeks, 101, 136
Legumes, 34, 120–121
Lemon, 67, 118–119, 170
Lentils, 34, 120–121
Lima beans, 65, 98
Limes, 119, 170
Live cultures, foods containing, 160
Liver detoxification, 59
Longevity, 23, 34, 60
Lunch, 33
Lycopene, 164

M
Maca root, 145
Macadamia nut, 122–123, 174
Mackerel, 159
Macronutrients, balancing
  intake of, 15

Magnesium, sources of, 26
Maitake mushrooms, 127
Maqui berries, 83
Matsutake mushrooms, 124
Meat, 34, 39
  grass-fed, 102–103
  healthier swaps for, 43
  myths about, 50
  recommended daily intake, 16
Medicine, food as, 11, 58
Memory, foods improving, 62
Metabolism, improving, 60
Milk, 148–149
Millet, 152
Mindful eating, 32–33
Mindfulness questions, about
  eating, 33
Mint, 181
Miso, 160
Mood, foods improving, 60, 62
Morris, Julie (author), 28–29
Mozzarella cheese, 84
Mulberries, 83
Multigrain bread, 56
Mushrooms, 34, 124–127
overcooking and, 65
recommended daily intake, 19
Mussels, 128–129
Myths about nutrition, debunked,
  46–53

N
"Natural," defined, 57
Navy beans, 120
Nectarines, 140
Nettle, 130–131
"Non-GMO," defined, 57
Northern white beans, 98
Nourishment, 21
Nut butters, 75
Nut oils, 135
Nutrient deficiency, 24–25
sources to replenish, 26–27

Nutrient-dense foods, 48
Nutrient density, 11
Nutrition boosting, ideas/methods
  for, 44–47
  deficient, 24–25
  improvement tips, 30–35
  myths debunked, 46–53
Nuts, 34, 60, 90, 172–175
  butters and oils, 75, 135
  recommended daily intake, 16

O
Oatmeal, 41
Oats, 76
Olive oil, 132–135
Omega-3 fatty acids, 22
Onions, 101, 136–137
recommended daily intake, 19
Oolong tea, 163
Oranges, 119, 181
Oregano, 156
Organic produce, 39, 138–139, 149
Overeating, 33, 52
Oyster mushrooms, 127
Oysters (shellfish), 66, 128–129

P
Parmesan cheese/crisps, 40, 84
Parsley root, 145
Pasta, 67
  healthier swap for, 41
"Pasture-raised," defined, 57
Peaches, 64, 140
Peanut butter, 75
Peanuts, 174
Peas. See Legumes
Pecans, 173, 174
Pecorino Romano cheese, 84
Phytochemicals, 14, 16
Pickled cabbage, 160–161
Pickles, 160
Pine nuts, 174
Pineapple, 67

Pistachios, 175
Plant-based diet, benefits of,
  20–23
Plums, 140–141
Poblano pepper, 112, 114
Popcorn, air-popped, 40
Poppy seeds, 107
Porcini mushrooms, 126
Pork, 102
Portion sizes, 33–34
Portobello mushrooms, 126
Potassium, sources of, 27
Potato chips, healthier swap for, 40
Potatoes, 142–143
Poultry, 102
Prediabetes, 61
Protein, 16
Pumpkin seed, 174
Pumpkin seed oil, 135
Pumpkin seeds, 107, 146–147
Purslane, 130

Q
Quantity, of food, 33–34
Quinoa, 150–151

R
Radish greens, 104
Radishes, 116, 145
Raspberries, 83, 96, 154–155
Raw milk, 149
Red peppers, benefit from, 60
Red/Red kidney beans, 79
Red wine, 60, 88
Reishi mushrooms, 127
Relaxation, foods promoting, 62
Resveratrol, 60
Rice
  diabetes and, 60
  healthier swap for, 41
Ricotta cheese, 85
Rooibos (red) tea, 163
Root vegetables, 144–145. See also

Potatoes
Rosemary, 156–157
Rutabaga, 116

S
Sacha inchi oil, 135
Sage, 156
Salmon, wild, 178–179
Salty/crunchy foods,
    healthier swaps for, 40
Sardines, 158–159, 179
Saturated (bad) fats, 51
Sauerkraut, 160–161
Scallions, 181
Scotch bonnet pepper, 112, 115
Sea Buckthorn, 83
Seafood, 34. See also individually
    named fish
Seaweed, 168–169
"Seconds," buying, 38
Seeds, 34, 174–175
    recommended daily intake, 16, 19
    wild rice, 176–177
Sesame seed oil, 107, 135
Sesame seeds, 107
Shallots, 101, 136
Shitake mushrooms, 124, 127
Shopping for food, tips on, 36–37
Shrimp, 67
Simple carbohydrates, 52
Skin, hair, and nails, 21
Skyr, 160, 182
Sleep, foods improving, 62
Slim Jim, healthier swap for, 43
Snacks, 33
Snickers bar, healthier swap for, 42
Soy sauce, 160
Spelt, 153
Spices, 33
Split peas, 120
Squash, 95. See also Zucchini/
    Zucchini noodles
Stone fruits, 140–141

Strawberries, 80, 82, 155
Stress, 61
Substitute foods, for healthier
    options, 40–43, 47
Sugary foods,
    healthier swaps for, 42
Summer squash. See Zucchini/
    Zucchini noodles
Sunflower seed oil, 107, 132, 135
Sunflower seeds, 107, 146, 175
Superfoods
    benefits of, 20–23
    concept of, 10
    incorporating into diet, 12
    Julie Morris on, 28–29
    nutrients in. See Nutrient entries;
    Nutrition
Swapping foods, for healthier
    options, 40–43, 47
Sweet foods,
    healthier swaps for, 42
Sweet potato, 143

T
Taste, 21, 46
Tea, 162–163
Teff, 153
Tempeh, 160
Thai (bird's eye) pepper, 115
Thyme, 156
Timing, of eating, 32–33
Tomatoes, 164–165
    growing your own, 38
Tubers, 144–145. See also Potatoes
Turkey jerky, 43
Turmeric, 124, 166–167
Turnip greens, 104
Turnips, 116
Type 2 diabetes, 60

U
Unsaturated (good) fats, 51
USDA (U.S. Department of

Agriculture)
    "certified organic," defined, 56–57
    nutrient deficiency and, 25
    recommended daily intake, 16

V
Vegetables, 34, 46
    in-season vs. frozen, 110–111
    organic, 39
    recommended daily intake, 15, 16
Veggie chips, 57
Vinegar, 170–171
Vitamin A, sources of, 27
Vitamin C, sources of, 27, 60
Vitamin D, sources of, 27
Vitamin E, sources of, 27

W
Walnut, 172–173
Wasabi, 108, 116
Wasted food, reducing, 38
Water, 88
Watercress, 116
Watermelon, 164
Weeds, 130–131
Weight gain/loss, 33, 58
White beans, 120
White Button mushrooms, 126
White tea, 163
Whole grains, 16, 34
Wild rice, 150, 176–177
Wild salmon, 178–179
Wood ear mushrooms, 124

Y
Yacón, 144
Yogurt, 160, 182–183
    frozen, 56

Z
Zest, citrus, 181
Zucchini/Zucchini noodles,
    41, 184–185

CREDITS

Shutterstock/bigacis; Shutterstock/Gregory Gerber; Shutterstock/Robyn Mackenzie; Shutterstock/bigacis **90-91** Getty Images/EyeEm **92-93** Getty Images/Westend61 **94-95** Alamy **96-97** Vladislav Nosick/Getty Images **98-99** Getty Images/iStockphoto; Moment/Getty Images **100-101** Getty Images/iStockphoto **102-103** Claudia Totir/ Getty Images **104-105** Shutterstock/chayun kajornkham; Shutterstock/K-Smile love; Shutterstock/Aleksandr Gogolin; yulkapopkova/Getty Images **106-107** Lew Robertson/Getty Images **108-109** StockFood/Getty Images; Shutterstock/ Yaruniv Studio **110-111** Getty Images/Dorling Kindersley **112-113** Getty Images/iStockphoto; Getty Images/Westend61 **114-115** Getty Images/ Tetra images; Shutterstock/nrazumov; Shutterstock/Judy Crawford; Shutterstock/pansticks; Shutterstock/Cabeca de Marmore; Shutterstock/Kara Grubis; Getty Images/Foodcollection **116-117** Getty Images/ iStockphoto **118-119** Shutterstock/Africa Studio **120-121** Claudia Totir/Getty Images **122-123** Shutterstock/Luis Echeverri Urrea **124-125** Shutterstock/kariphoto; Shutterstock/Wealthylady; Shutterstock/Nishihama; Getty Images/iStockphoto; Getty Images/Foodcollection **126-127** Siri Stafford/Getty Images; Getty Images/Mixa; Shutterstock/3DE Studios; Shutterstock/schankz; Shutterstock/vinbergv; Erica McCaig/Getty Images; Shutterstock/kristof lauwers; Shutterstock/12photography; Shutterstock/Jiang Zhongyan **128-129** Eugene Mymrin/Getty Images **130-131** Shutterstock/ Julia Sudnitskaya **132-133** EyeEm/Getty Images **134-135** MARKA/Alamy **136-137** Busakorn Pongparnit/Getty Images **138-139** Getty Images/Foodcollection **140-141** Verdina Anna/Gety Images **142-143** Shutterstock/Sea Wave **144-145** Shuttersto/Jiang Hongyan; Shutterstock/Nattika; AlasdairJames/Getty Images; Shutterstock/Kaiskynet Studio; Shutterstock/Maks Narodenko; Shutterstock/Anna Kucherova; Shutterstock/Yossi James **146-147** Natalya Danko/EyeEm/ Getty Images **148-149** Shutterstock/Africa Studio **150-151** Shutterstock/Foxys Forest Manufacture **152-153** Shutterstock/ picturepartners; E+/Getty Images; Shutterstock/Moving Moment; Shutterstock/Rtstudio; Paolo Negri/Getty Images; Shutterstock / Elizabeth A.Cummings; Getty Images/Foodcollection **154-155** Prostock-Studio/Getty Images **156** Shutterstock/mr.chanwit wangsuk **157** Shutterstock/Nataliya Arzamasova **158-159** twomeows/Getty Images **160-161** Getty Images/Westend61 **162-163** E+/Getty Images; Roman Tsubin/Getty Images; Getty Images/500px; Getty Images/iStockphoto **164-165** Getty Images/Alloy **166-167** MAIKA 777/Getty Images; Shutterstock/sama_ja **168-169** Westend61/Getty Images; Shutterstock/akepong srichaichana **170-171** E+/Getty Images **172-173** E+/Getty Images **174-175** James Baigrie/Getty Images; Kazuo Ogawa/Getty Images; James Baigrie/Getty Images; William Turner/Getty Images; Juanmonino/Getty Images; Yvonne Duivenvoorden/Getty Images; David Bishop/Getty Images; AYImages/Getty Images; James Baigrie/Getty Images; David Murray/Getty Images; kodiak/Getty Images; James Baigrie/Getty Images; James Baigrie/Getty Images **176-177** Shutterstock/Stolyevych Yuliya **178-179** Eugene Mymrin/Getty Images **180** Westend61/Getty Images **181** Shutterstock/AleksandraN; Shutterstock/Sea Wave; Shutterstock/Fascinadora; Shutterstock/ArtemSh **182-183** Getty Images/iStockphoto **184-185** Shutterstock/SunKids

SPECIAL THANKS TO CONTRIBUTING WRITERS:
Susan Barkman, Beth Johnson, Anne Marie O'Connor, Philip C. Price

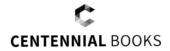

CENTENNIAL BOOKS

An Imprint of
Centennial Media, LLC
40 Worth St., 10th Floor
New York, NY 10013, U.S.A.

CENTENNIAL BOOKS is a trademark of Centennial Media, LLC

ISBN 978-1-951274-17-7

Distributed by
Simon & Schuster, Inc.
1230 Avenue of the Americas
New York, NY 10020, U.S.A.

For information about custom editions, special sales and premium and corporate purchases,
please contact Centennial Media at contact@centennialmedia.com.

Manufactured in China

Publishers & Co-Founders Ben Harris, Sebastian Raatz
Editorial Director Annabel Vered
Creative Director Jessica Power
Executive Editor Janet Giovanelli
Deputy Editor Alyssa Shaffer
Design Director Ben Margherita
Senior Art Director Laurene Chavez
Art Directors Natali Suasnavas, Joseph Ulatowski
Production Manager Paul Rodina
Production Assistant Alyssa Swiderski
Editorial Assistant Tiana Schippa
Sales & Marketing Jeremy Nurnberg